Alternative Therapies

ISSUES

Volume 81

Editor

Craig Donnellan

Independence

Educational Publishers

First published by Independence
PO Box 295
Cambridge CB1 3XP
England

British Library Cataloguing in Publication Data
Alternative Therapies – (Issues Series)
I. Donnellan, Craig II. Series
615.5

ISBN 1 86168 276 X

Printed in Great Britain
MWL Print Group Ltd

Typeset by
Claire Boyd

Cover
The illustration on the front cover is by
Pumpkin House.

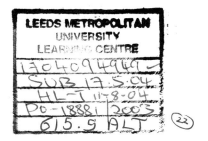

CONTENTS

Introduction

Alternative Therapies is the eighty-first volume in the **Issues** series. The aim of this series is to offer up-to-date information about important issues in our world.

Alternative Therapies looks at the various types of complementary and alternative therapies and the medical debate.

The information comes from a wide variety of sources and includes:
Government reports and statistics
Newspaper reports and features
Magazine articles and surveys
Web site material
Literature from lobby groups
and charitable organisations.

It is hoped that, as you read about the many aspects of the issues explored in this book, you will critically evaluate the information presented. It is important that you decide whether you are being presented with facts or opinions. Does the writer give a biased or an unbiased report? If an opinion is being expressed, do you agree with the writer?

Alternative Therapies offers a useful starting-point for those who need convenient access to information about the many issues involved. However, it is only a starting-point. At the back of the book is a list of organisations which you may want to contact for further information.

*****

What is complementary medicine?

Information from the Institute for Complementary Medicine

Complementary Medicine (CM) includes many different techniques of treating a patient. These are based on systems practised thousands of years ago and can in fact be considered to be the original forms of medicine. They all have one aspect in common which is that they treat the patient as a whole person rather than treating a specific symptom or symptoms. They do this by treating the life force of the patient at their physical, mental and emotional levels.

Some people used to refer to CM as 'Fringe' or 'Alternative' because they consider it to be alternative to the 'Allopathic Medicine' that is practised by the General Medical Practitioners (GPs). But CM *complements* the needs of the patient and is a more accurate description as this term describes the methods of healing that treat the complete or whole person. Hence 'Complementary Medicine' is the most appropriate title.

Below is a glossary of some of the many disciplines within Complementary Medicine in alphabetical order:

Acupressure
Using the acupuncture points, pressure from the fingers is applied where appropriate.

Acupuncture
Fine needles are inserted into the body at meridians or energy centres. This 'unblocks' or regulates the CHI energy circulating the body, which, in turn, stimulates the healing process. There is a mass of Chinese research but Western science does not yet accept the principle.

Alexander Technique
F. M. Alexander (1896-1955) was an Australian actor who lost his voice. He realigned his posture and found the voice returned. The Technique is to persuade the body to return to its normal position and so allow the brain to recognise and retain the realignment. The head and neck positioning are particularly important.

Auricular Acupuncture
The ear has a number of meridian points and can be used to affect the whole body. There has been some research using this method of treatment for drug addiction.

Bach Flowers
These formulae were developed by Dr Bach as an offshoot of homeopathic medicine. The usefulness of this lies in the way the remedies can

---

Complementary Medicine (CM) includes many different techniques of treating a patient

---

be effective treatment of mood swings and emotional conditions. The remedy for shock and other upsets is considered particularly helpful.

Biodynamic Massage
In common with all Complementary Medical treatments, the vital force is perceived to affect all the organs of the body. The link between the psyche and the physical was further developed by Gerda Boyesen in the Norwegian hospital service in the late 1960s, where she used massage to remove emotional trauma from organs of the body. She claimed to detect the variations in health by monitoring the fluid sounds through her stethoscope.

Chiropractic
Manipulation of the spine and movement of the extremities attributed to D.D. Palmer about 1890. Chiropractors vary in their approach. Some give extended massage before treatment whilst others do not.

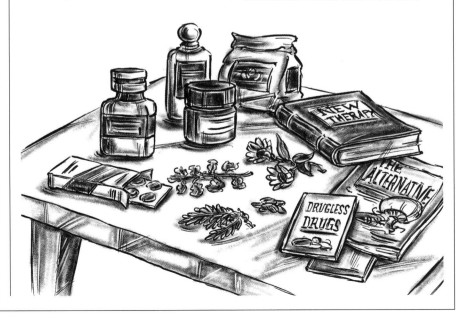

Chinese Medicine

Has much in common with other Eastern systems and is the foundation of many techniques currently used in the West. Provides a comprehensive range of treatments for problems arising from imbalances at physical, mental, emotional and spiritual parts of the consciousness.

Colour Therapy

The benefits of coloured light on the skin are well known and the colour practitioner will diagnose and provide the appropriate coloured light to help bring back health and well-being. There are other systems such as:

Detecting the colours in the energy field of the individual and providing the tints which will help achieve a return to the normal. This is often practised by healers with the gift of extended perception either by sight or touch.

Colour can be used in the choice of clothing and furnishing since they affect the mood and attitude of mind.

Cranial Osteopathy

Developed by Dr William Sutherland in the 1930s, as an extension of the ancient Chinese Tuina and Osteopathic techniques. The process appears to rely on the practitioner's healing energies directed into the head and neck. Practitioners claim to feel a slight movement in the bones of the skull which sceptics claim is not possible.

Crystal Healing

Crystals transmit energy which are claimed to be able to tune to the body's fluctuating vibrations. Crystals are chosen according to their energy and the needs of the patient.

Flotation

Floating in water in a darkened pool amounts to sensory deprivation and this can trigger healing. The support of the water, which often contains Epsom salts, can rest injuries and help the patient to achieve good balance between the left and right cortex of the brain.

Herbal Medicine

Herbs are used in both Eastern and Western medicine. The aim is to use

all parts of the herb and particular emphasis is laid on the energetic content of the herb and its ability to stimulate healing.

Thus the method of picking the herb and the time of day can affect the potency. The whole herb has a wider healing potential than the single active agent used by the pharmaceutical industry.

Holism

Generally regarded as a word from HOLOS – Greek for whole. In Complementary Medicine the whole is seen as more than the sum of the parts and describes treatments which are focused on the physical, mental, emotions, vital force, Spirit and Soul.

Homeopathy

Hippocrates and Samual Hahnemann (1796) are credited with using the homeopathic principle. This means treating the vital force to enable the body to re-energise its own repair mechanisms. The homeopathic remedy does not treat the presenting symptom but the body's ability to heal itself with the result that prescriptions for the same named disease will probably be different in each case.

Hydrotherapy

Bathing in water has been used throughout history but the mineral baths which were opened during the nineteenth century in the UK and Europe claimed the most successful treatments.

Hypnotherapy

This is not just hypnosis but a partnership between practitioner and patient which aims at defining the cause of the problem thereby helping the patient to overcome it in their own way and a time scale of their choice.

Iridology

Diagnosis from the iris of the eye which is the exposed nerve endings which are seen as the coloured area. There is little reliable research but qualified practitioners appear able to make a significant contribution to helping the patient to understand those parts of the body which need attention.

Kinesiology

The use of testing muscle strength to find products which disturb the patient's well-being. Can be used to find which foods are most conducive to health and those which may cause unwanted symptoms. It is also used to find the appropriate natural medicine such as a homeopathic remedy.

Manipulative Medicine

Based on massage techniques and structural manipulation.

When used in the ancient Chinese way, the whole emphasis is on gentleness and encouraging the muscles to relax before attempting to help to re-align the bones. Attempting to make adjustments before this relaxation has been completed can result in considerable pain and the change may well not be permanent. In these cases, many treatments will be required which is not the case when the preliminary work is correctly completed.

Naturopathy

The naturopath will have many different treatments to offer but all are based on the concept that the body will heal itself if given the right stimulus.

Nutritional Therapy

The diet can have dramatic influences on our health and well-being. If we recognise that the body chemistry of each person is different, the need for different diets is apparent.

Osteopathy

Structure governs function is the tenet of osteopathy. Andrew Taylor Still is given credit for initiating the system at the end of the American Civil War but there is much in common with chiropractic and the

Eastern techniques of ensuring that the skeleton is in correct alignment so that nerves are not pinched.

Oxygen Therapy
Forms of oxygen (ozone) have been used in many contexts from water purification to a disinfectant in the bottling industry. As a treatment, it has been recognised that harmful bacteria and viruses can only live in a low oxygen environment. Treatments vary from sitting in a 'steam' bath and being surrounded by ozone to treating the blood by passing ozone through it and clearing impurities. Dr Otto Warburg proved that cancer cannot live in a high oxygen environment.

Pilates
Specific exercises to correct the posture first developed by Joseph Pilates in the USA. Now available in the UK.

Qi Gong
Part of Traditional Chinese Medicine. Means energy practice and involves the transmission of the healing energy into the patient.

Reflexology
The principle is that all the organs in the body are reflected on the foot or hand. By pressing the relevant point, healing can be transferred to the particular area in need. Original practitioners thought that crystal of lactic acid which caused sensitivity must be crushed to enable healing to take place. The pain was often considerable and this process has been superseded with more gentle methods.

Reflex Touch
This is a development associated with Patricia Morrell who achieved success with her methods of diagnosis and light touch (Morrell Reflexology) which have been further refined.

Reiki
A Japanese healing discipline developed by Mikao Usui. The principles are similar to most other healing techniques except that the system follows a pre-determined set of hand positions which form the basis for each treatment. The system replies on the development of the student's ability to transfer the healing energy and this may take considerable time. Some courses offer a mastership in three weekends.

Shiatsu
A Japanese system similar to acupuncture without the needles. The practitioner may use elbows, feet, knees and fingers to transfer the QI or vital energy to balance the whole body of the patient.

Sports Massage
Particular treatments aimed at maintaining the strength and muscle power of the sports person. Emphasis is usually on prevention.

Swedish Massage
Common system of massage using kneading, stroking and pummelling to achieve relaxation and increased circulation of the blood.

Tai Chi
Part of Traditional Chinese Medicine. Flowing slow movement and breathing techniques stimulate and regulate the flow of Chi energy.

Traditional Chinese Medicine
The basis of much ancient healing wisdom which also shows a similarity to other traditional medicine in both thought and delivery of treatment. The belief stems from the concept of Yin and Yang – Yin being about the feminine traits, quiet calm and intro-spection whilst Yang represents loud-ness, light and masculine traits. These must be balanced to achieve health and well-being. Treatments include exercise and manipulation (Tuina), herbal medicines, healing (Qi Gong) and acupressure amongst others.

Yoga
Indian medicine places much emphasis on prevention and yoga is used with that in mind. There are many different types of yoga postural and stretching exercises and the student is always advised to go to a qualified teacher.

■ The above article is an extract of information from the Institute for Complementary Medicine. For a full listing of complementary medicines visit their web site at www.icmedicine.co.uk

© Institute for Complementary Medicine (ICM)

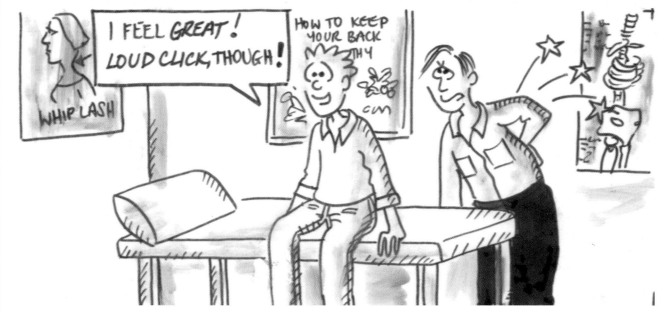

What is natural medicine?

Information from *Saga Magazine*

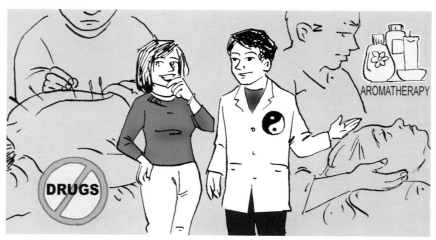

Natural, complementary and alternative all mean much the same thing when it comes to medicine in that they treat the whole person.

Natural medicine is an umbrella term that includes an enormous range of approaches from aromatherapy to visualisation. You could think of it as any health-enhancing therapy that does not involve taking orthodox medication, surgery or conventional treatment such as physiotherapy. As a rule, it is not available on the NHS, although some GPs and hospital departments now provide or arrange for patients to be offered treatments such as homeopathy, osteopathy, chiropractic and aromatherapy.

This article provides information on what is often called 'complementary' or 'alternative' medicine. In fact, most practitioners in the UK prefer the term complementary medicine because they do not regard their treatment as an alternative to that offered by the medical profession. Complementary therapy is intended to work in parallel with any conventional treatment you may be receiving and not to replace it.

Practitioners of complementary medicine claim that one of the main differences between them and most members of the medical profession is that they treat the whole person rather than just any disease or symptoms they may have. In other words, their approach is holistic. This means that your first consultation with a complementary therapist will be mostly (or entirely) taken up with an extended question-and-answer session covering all aspects of your lifestyle as well as your medical history and any current symptoms or problems.

It is worth bearing in mind that most complementary medicine aims to promote overall wellbeing and positive health; it does not confine itself exclusively to alleviating symptoms or treating existing illnesses. Even if you are not actually unwell or if you have a condition that cannot be cured, complementary therapy may have something to offer you.

If you are being treated by your doctor for an existing condition, it is wise to tell him or her when you are planning to try some form of complementary therapy in case there is some good reason why this would not be advisable. For example, massage may not be suitable for those with some forms of arthritis or cancer; herbal medicine may react adversely with certain prescribed medications. While many doctors are sceptical of the benefits of complementary medicine, others are more open-minded. Even if your doctor is dubious, you can still go ahead provided he or she does not have a sound medical reason for objecting.

Choosing a therapy

Some therapies are particularly helpful for certain symptoms and conditions: for example, osteopathy and chiropractic for back pain, massage for muscle and other soft tissue damage, aromatherapy, meditation and relaxation for stress. However, it is important that you feel comfortable with a therapy and with the individual therapist if you are to gain any benefit. For example, if you dislike the prospect of undressing before a stranger, you might prefer acupressure or reflexology to massage; if you are of a practical turn of mind, you might find osteopathy more acceptable than reiki or visualisation.

Before you start

Once you have made your choice of therapy, you need to ensure that the therapist you plan to consult has appropriate qualifications and experience and find out whether their approach is likely to be right for you. A reputable practitioner will be happy to answer your questions and will not encourage you to have treatment if it is unlikely to do you any good. Be wary of anyone who offers to cure you when orthodox medicine cannot do so and try to be realistic about what can and can't be achieved. Questions you might consider asking include:

- What training and qualifications does the therapist have?
- Do they belong to a professional organisation?
- Do you feel comfortable with the therapist and his or her approach?
- Is this therapy safe for me?
- How will I benefit from this treatment?
- How many sessions will I need?
- How frequent will the sessions be?
- How many people has this therapist treated with my condition/symptoms and with what results?
- How much will a course of treatment cost?

© *Saga Magazine*

About acupuncture

Information from the British Medical Acupuncture Society (BMAS)

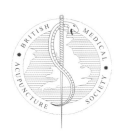

What is the BMAS?

Acupuncture is a medical technique used to treat a wide variety of conditions.

The British Medical Acupuncture Society is a nationwide group of family doctors and hospital specialists who practise acupuncture alongside more conventional techniques. The BMAS believes that acupuncture has an important role to play in health care today.

During the past few years, acupuncture has become increasingly popular. Whilst it is exciting that the range of medical applications of acupuncture is increasing, it does mean that the responsible practitioner of acupuncture has a duty to educate both other medical colleagues and the general public about the strengths and weaknesses of the technique.

Very large claims have been made for acupuncture in the past. Not all of them can be substantiated. Such claims are worrying and can alienate many people – doctors among them – who might otherwise be sympathetic to the view that acupuncture can, in selected cases, be an effective method of treatment.

In this article, the BMAS has provided detailed information to help you decide whether acupuncture might be a useful treatment to try for your condition. We also provide information to help you select an appropriate practitioner.

What is acupuncture?

Acupuncture is a treatment which can relieve symptoms of some physical and psychological conditions and may encourage the patient's body to heal and repair itself, if it is able to do so.

Acupuncture stimulates the nerves in skin and muscle, and can produce a variety of effects. We know that it increases the body's release of natural painkillers – endorphin and serotonin – in the pain pathways of both the spinal cord and the brain.

This modifies the way pain signals are received.

But acupuncture does much more than reduce pain, and has a beneficial effect on health. Patients often notice an improved sense of well-being after treatment.

Modern research shows that acupuncture can affect most of the body's systems – the nervous system, muscle tone, hormone outputs, circulation, antibody production and allergic responses, as well as the respiratory, digestive, urinary, and reproductive systems.

Each patient's case will be assessed by the practitioner and treatment will be tailored to the individual; so it is impossible to give more than a general idea of what treatment might involve. Typically, fine needles are inserted through the skin and left in position briefly, sometimes with manual or electrical stimulation. The number of needles varies but may be only two or three. Treatment might be once a week to begin with, then at longer intervals as the condition responds. A typical course of treatment lasts 5 to 8 sessions.

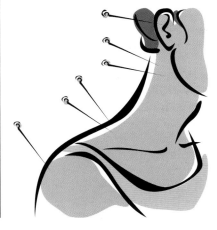

Uses for acupuncture

Taking the above into consideration, here are some of the ways in which acupuncture may be effective:

- Pain relief for a wide range of painful conditions.
- It is commonly used to treat musculoskeletal pain, for example back, shoulder, neck and leg pain.
- It has been used successfully to treat headaches, migraines, trapped nerves, chronic muscle strains, sports injuries and various kinds of arthritic and rheumatic pain.
- Functional bowel or bladder problems such as IBS or even mild forms of incontinence.
- Menstrual and menopausal symptoms, e.g. period pains and hot flushes.
- Allergies such as hay fever, perennial allergic rhinitis, and some types of allergic rashes such as urticaria and prickly heat.
- Some other skin problems such as rashes and ulcers, itching, some forms of dermatitis and some cases of excessive sweating.
- Sinus problems and chronic catarrh. Dry mouth and eyes.
- Help with stopping smoking.

This list is by no means exhaustive, but it does give a rough idea of the wide range of conditions that respond to acupuncture treatment. Remember that before starting acupuncture, the practitioner must be sure of the diagnosis and that all the necessary tests have been carried out which might point to any serious or potentially serious condition, perhaps requiring other forms of treatment.

Acupuncture – past, present and future

Acupuncture-like techniques have been used for over 5,000 years. A comprehensive system was developed in the Far East and this was first introduced into Europe in the 17th century. However, widespread interest in the technique did not develop until the political events of the early 1970s allowed travel restrictions between East and West to be eased.

In the past thirty years, because of the huge public interest in the subject, considerable scientific research on acupuncture has been carried out – although much remains to be done. We now know much more about how acupuncture works and some of the myths can be laid to rest. It is demonstrably untrue to say that the results of acupuncture are all in the mind.

As we learn more about it, the possibilities of using acupuncture alongside orthodox medicine increase. The distinction between complementary or alternative medicine and conventional medicine is becoming blurred as acupuncture is accepted in medicine. Acupuncture is already available in most hospital pain clinics and it is provided by an ever-increasing number of GPs and hospital doctors.

Where to go for acupuncture

At the moment, anybody in the UK is allowed to call themselves doctor or acupuncturist and can start advertising and practising acupuncture immediately, regardless of qualifications or experience. This is deeply worrying to the British Medical Acupuncture Society whose members are all registered medical practitioners with long experience of medicine.

Our members are subject to our Code of Practice and Complaints Procedure in addition to regulation by the General Medical Council.

Acupuncture is a potent therapy, and whilst it is generally safer than most conventional treatments, if used without due care it can have serious adverse effects and interactions with other treatments.

Acupuncture should only be used by trained practitioners who can adequately assess the risks and benefits of applying the therapy.

The ideal promoted by the BMAS is that acupuncture should be fully incorporated into orthodox medicine and used as one of the therapeutic tools available in treatment of a defined range of conditions. Clearly a GP or hospital doctor who is trained in the use of acupuncture can do this, but safe and considered therapy may be available from a non-medical practitioner who works in close communication and co-operation with a patient's regular medical attendant.

How to find a practitioner

Your family doctor, local Primary Care Organisation or local Health Authority may be able to tell you the name of your nearest medical acupuncturist.

■ The above information is from the British Medical Acupuncture Society's web site which can be found at www.medical-acupuncture.org.uk
© The British Medical Acupuncture Society

Osteopathy in the UK

Your questions answered by the General Osteopathic Council

What is osteopathy?
Osteopathy is an established recognised system of diagnosis and treatment, which lays its main emphasis on the structural and functional integrity of the body. It is distinctive by the fact that it recognises that much of the pain and disability which we suffer stems from abnormalities in the function of the body structure as well as damage caused to it by disease.

[Description by General Osteopathic Council, 28 October 1998]

What kinds of problems can osteopathy help with?
Whilst back pain is the most common problem seen, osteopathy can help with a wide variety of problems including changes to posture in pregnancy, babies with colic or sleeplessness, repetitive strain injury, postural problems caused by driving or work strain, children with glue

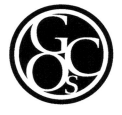

ear, the pain of arthritis and sports injuries among many others. Leaflets explaining many of the common treatments used are available from the Osteopathic Information Service.

Your local Registered Osteopath will be happy to advise as to whether they could help with your own particular problem.

What can I expect when I visit an osteopath?
When you visit an osteopath for the first time a full case history will be taken and you will be given an examination. You will normally be asked to remove some of your clothing and to perform a simple series of movements. The osteopath will then use a highly developed sense of touch, called palpation, to identify any points of weakness or excessive strain throughout the body.

The osteopath may need additional investigations such as x-ray or blood tests. This will allow a full diagnosis and suitable treatment plan to be developed for you.

How much do treatments cost?
Treatments are approximately £20-£30 for a 30-40-minute treatment session. Often the first session is longer and may cost more.

How many treatments will I need?
Osteopathy is patient centred, which means treatment is geared to you as an individual. Your osteopath should be able to give you an indication after your first visit. For some acute pain one or two treatments may be

all that is necessary. Chronic conditions may need ongoing maintenance. An average is 6-8 sessions.

Do I need a referral from my GP?
A formal referral from your GP is not necessary, the majority of osteopathic patients self-refer.

How does osteopathy work?
Osteopaths work with their hands using a wide variety of treatment techniques. These may include soft tissue techniques, rhythmic passive joint mobilisation or the high velocity thrust techniques designed to improve mobility and the range of movement of a joint. Gentle release techniques are widely used, particularly when treating children or elderly patients. This allows the body to return to efficient normal function.

How can I be sure I am in safe hands when visiting an osteopath?
A Registered Osteopath has demonstrated to the General Osteopathic Council that they meet the highest standards of safety and competency. Proof of good health, good character and professional indemnity insurance is also a requirement.

I have noticed many osteopaths have the letters DO and/or BSc(Ost) after their names, what does this mean?
These are osteopathic qualifications. The DO stands for diploma in osteopathy and the BSc is a degree in osteopathy. Both qualifications hold equal status except that the diploma has been replaced by degree courses validated by universities.

Can I have osteopathic treatment on the NHS?
Most people consult an osteopath privately. Telephone local practices to find out about fees in your area. An increasing number of osteopaths work with GP practices and commissioning authorities so that it may be possible for your doctor to refer you to an osteopath on the NHS

Can I have osteopathy on my private medical insurance?
Many private health insurance schemes give benefit for osteopathic treatment. Some companies will reimburse the total fee or pay a

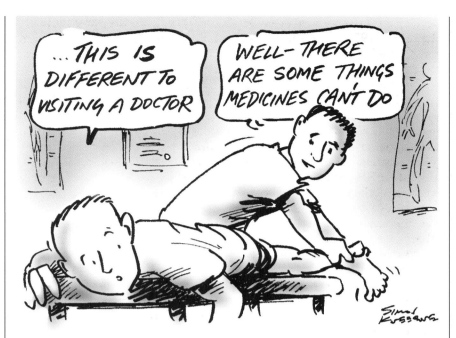

percentage of the costs. Contact the helpline of your insurance company who will explain the actual benefits and methods of claim for your individual policy.

What should I do if I am unhappy with my osteopathic treatment?
Often problems are caused by misunderstandings and can easily be resolved by discussing your concerns with the osteopath directly. If this does not resolve the problem or your concerns are of a more serious nature the GOsC has a Code of Practice which patients may refer to.

What is the status of osteopathy in the UK?
Osteopaths are statutorily regulated health professionals and form an integral part of primary care teams.

More on statutory regulation
It is a criminal offence in the UK, liable to prosecution, to describe oneself as an osteopath unless registered with the General Osteopathic Council. The General Osteopathic Council regulates, promotes and develops the profession of osteopathy, maintaining a Statutory Register of those entitled to practise osteopathy.

How do I find a Registered Osteopath?
Our online searchable database can help find a locally Registered Osteopath.

What are the origins of osteopathy?
Andrew Taylor Still, born in 1828 in Virginia, USA, trained as a doctor according to the system of medical education available at the time. As time went on he followed a different path from many of his peers, eschewing alcohol and the habit of contemporary physicians of administering crude drugs at their disposal in heroic quantities. This drove him to seek new methods of treating sickness. The outcome of his research was the application of physical treatment as a specialised form of treatment for which he coined the name 'Osteopathy'.

In 1892 A. T. Still organised a school in Kirksville, Missouri, for the teaching of osteopathy and it was from these small beginnings that osteopathy was brought to the UK around the turn of the century. The first school of osteopathy in the UK was set in London in 1917 and over time other schools and colleges followed.

Today there are around 3,000 osteopaths in the UK performing over six million patient consultations a year.

How do I become an osteopath?
For details of training to become an osteopath see our web site.

■ The above information is from the General Osteopathic Council's web site which can be found at www.osteopathy.org.uk
© General Osteopathic Council

Chiropractic

Information from the British Chiropractic Association

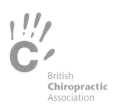

British
Chiropractic
Association

What is chiropractic?

Chiropractors treat problems with your joints, bones and muscles, and the effects they have on your nervous system. Working on all the joints of your body, concentrating particularly on the spine, they use their hands to make often gentle, specific adjustments (the chiropractic word for manipulation) to improve the efficiency of your nervous system and release your body's natural healing ability. Chiropractic does not involve the use of any drugs or surgery.

Members of the British Chiropractic Association (BCA) abide by a strict code of ethics and the association only accepts members who have graduated from a nationally or internationally recognised college of chiropractic education after a minimum of four years' full-time training. The BCA ensures its chiropractors maintain high standards of conduct, practice, education and training. Like medical practitioners and dentists, all chiropractors are registered by law.

Your first visit

Will treatment hurt?

Generally, a chiropractic adjustment does not hurt – although there may be some minor short-term discomfort which quickly passes for most patients. You will normally find that follow-up treatments are much more pleasant, as your symptoms improve and you feel more at ease with your chiropractor.

Are there any risks?

Chiropractic has far fewer risks than many other treatments for your problem. Serious side effects are extremely uncommon. Very rarely, manipulation of the neck has been linked with strokes, although research shows that chiropractic is one of the safest and most effective forms of treatment available. Your BCA chiropractor will, of course, be happy to discuss all your concerns regarding treatment.

Chiropractors treat problems with your joints, bones and muscles, and the effects they have on your nervous system

---

Do chiropractors use X-rays?

Any decision to take X-rays will be made in consultation with you. At all times, your BCA chiropractor will weigh the risks against the benefits and advise you accordingly. Typical circumstances where an X-ray may be necessary are recent injuries, older patients whose bone structure may have altered over time, unusual examination findings or a history of serious diseases.

Servicing your spine

How often should check-ups be given?

Chiropractors practise in two main ways: one is to minimise the recurrence of your pain through 'supportive care'. The practitioner may recommend a check-up every two to six months depending on your original complaint and your lifestyle. The other approach is known as 'wellness care'. Here, the chiropractor may wish to check you more frequently, as well as exploring with you further ways you can enhance your wellbeing.

Aren't good diet and exercise enough?

They certainly help, but cannot always deal with an existing problem in the same way as chiropractic. This is because where exercise can

---

Categories of complementary and alternative medicine (CAM) disciplines

Group One Professionally organised alternative therapies	Group Two Complementary therapies	Group Three Alternative disciplines
Acupuncture	Alexander technique	**3a: Long-established and traditional systems of health care:**
Chiropractic	Aromatherapy	
Herbal medicine	Bach and other flower remedies	
Homeopathy	Massage	Ayurvedic medicine
Osteopathy	Reflexology	Anthroposophical medicine
	Healing including Reiki	Chinese herbal medicine
	Hypnotherapy	Traditional Chinese medicine
	Shiatsu	**3b: Other alternative disciplines**
		Crystal therapy
		Dowsing
		Iridology
		Kinesiology
		Radionics

Source: House of Lords Select Committee Report, 2000

improve the overall fitness of your body, chiropractic can target the individual problem areas that are reducing its efficiency.

Isn't too much chiropractic bad?
Your BCA chiropractor is trained and qualified to diagnose your problem, evaluate when it is appropriate to give treatment and, in particular, when not to. Your case will be assessed on an individual basis. However – no one should become dependent on any one treatment. If you have concerns, please discuss your treatment plan with your chiropractor.

Back pain
Is it a slipped disc?
Spinal discs are fibrous rings, containing a soft gel-like 'cushion', between each of your spinal bones (vertebrae). Discs cannot slip, because they are attached to the vertebrae, but the term 'slipped disc' can mean disc damage such as a bulge, a tear or a partial or total collapse. The resulting pressure on the nerves that come out of your spine can cause pain in your back, or 'referred' pain in the area to which the nerves branch out. Sciatica, for example, is leg pain caused by nerve pressure in the lower spine. Your BCA chiropractor will explain the cause of your pain – it may not be a slipped disc, as this term can be overused.

How long will chiropractic take to work?
Guidelines for medical practitioners state that spinal manipulation can help back pain, especially if carried out within the first six weeks. The longer you have been in pain, the longer it will take to heal. Your chiropractor will advise you of your likely recovery time, and how to minimise the chances of the problem happening again. Early treatment is important but chiropractors are also effective at treating long-standing or chronic pain

Is chiropractic treatment possible after surgery?
Probably. Your chiropractor has the training and experience to treat

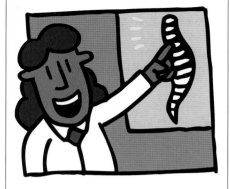

each patient as an individual. You will receive appropriate treatment and adjustments for your specific condition, while areas not suitable for treatment will be carefully avoided. Many chiropractors are able to offer post-surgical exercise, advice and rehabilitation.

Save your neck
Is it safe to adjust the neck?
Yes, 66-69% of visits to a chiropractor include cervical (neck) adjustments. Recent publications suggest that chiropractic treatment to be extremely safe, when carried out by a skilled individual.

How about wearing a collar ?
Although in the acute stage a soft collar may be worn for a short time, collars should not be relied upon. If you become reliant on a collar, the muscles of your neck will become weaker as their job is being done by the collar. It is important, therefore, to have an active treatment plan that involves your chiropractor, ergonomic advice and possibly an exercise programme to help support the muscles and joints of your neck.

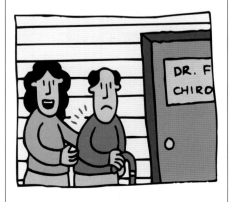

Is rolling your head good for your neck?
No. Many people in the past have been given neck or head rolling exercises to help stretch their necks. However, the joints in your neck are really designed for single movements like turning or looking up, down, left or right – not all of these movements together. A safer exercise may be just to do each of these movements individually.

Wear and tear
What about just taking painkillers or anti-inflammatory drugs?
These can dull your pain, but it may well return as they do not necessarily deal with the cause. They may also have side effects.

How can chiropractic help joints that are already degenerated?
Degenerated joints are sometimes the result of the surrounding joints not doing their fair share of work, so that the load is not managed equally. Chiropractic aims to restore your normal joint function spreading the load and taking excessive strain away from degenerated joints. Your BCA chiropractors can also give you advice on exercise for maintaining joint function.

Can chiropractors help osteoporosis?
Osteoporosis happens when the amount of calcium in the bones (which gives them strength) is very low and leaves them weak and easily breakable. This is particularly common in women past the menopause. However, having osteoporosis doesn't mean that you will have a fracture. Your BCA chiropractor will be able to use various modified treatment methods to cater for someone with osteoporosis as well as advise on other available treatments. Chiropractic helps to keep your joints mobile and improve your balance and muscle tone to minimise the risk of falling.

■ The above information is from the British Chiropractic Association's web site which can be found at www.chiropractic-uk.co.uk Alternatively see their address details on page 41.

Professional aromatherapy

A brief guide from the IFPA, the aromatherapy specific organisation

What is aromatherapy?

Aromatherapy is the therapeutic use of essential oils to relieve nervous stress, enhance wellbeing, and promote health and vitality.

Essential oils are highly fragrant, volatile (quickly evaporating) fluids that occur naturally in aromatic plants growing the world over. They can be distilled from flowers, leaves, seeds, roots, fruits and woods, depending upon the plant. Essential oils that are commonly used in aromatherapy include lavender, geranium, bergamot, clary sage and rose.

Where does aromatherapy come from?

Essential oils have been used in perfumery, food flavouring and medicine for about a thousand years. Long before they were first distilled in Persia, the ancient Egyptians produced scented oils from frankincense, cedarwood and other plants – utilised by priests and perfumers alike.

However, the word 'aromatherapie' was coined as recently as 1928 – by French chemist Rene-Maurice Gattefosse.

Initially, aromatherapy gained popularity in the UK as a beauty treatment; however, the increasing recognition of its therapeutic potential by orthodox health care professionals has made it one of our fastest-growing complementary therapies.

How does aromatherapy work?

Each essential oil has distinct therapeutic properties that improve the body's natural functioning and so help to prevent disease. Enhancing the health of both mind and body, they have been shown through research to possess stimulant, anti-infectious, anti-inflammatory and relaxant properties, among others.

The ability of essential oils to have a psychologically calming or uplifting effect is directly linked to

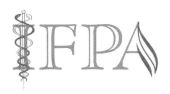

the influence of their wonderful aromas – one that depends on the close link between olfaction (smelling) and the brain.

During aromatherapy massage the aroma of the essential oils calms the mind and relaxes the nervous system. The stress-relieving effect of the treatment encourages us to use our mental energy more productively. Relaxed and refreshed, we are able to face life's challenges with a renewed sense of confidence.

In the professional practice of aromatherapy, essential oils are applied in a variety of ways including massage, ointments, lotions, baths and inhalations. Their holistic application is geared towards the needs of the individual. Aromatherapists appreciate the fact that each individual requires a unique blend of essences.

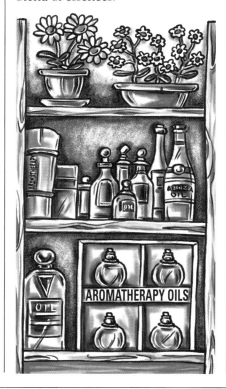

Combining the benefits of essential oils with those of therapeutic massage produces a pleasurable yet effective method of healing. Together, they enhance the circulation of blood and lymph, relax and tone tense, tired muscles, and promote a sense of overall well being.

Is aromatherapy safe?

Essential oils are naturally highly concentrated and must be diluted before being applied. For use in massage they are mixed with a carrier such as almond, walnut or sunflower oil. Massage is one of the safest ways for the body to benefit from plant essences, as the skin absorbs oil rather slowly.

Essential oils are, however, very powerful, and so should always be used with care – preferably under the guidance of a professionally trained aromatherapist.

Can anyone benefit from aromatherapy?

Aromatherapy can be of benefit to everyone – whether his or her health is good or requires improvement. It is used to relieve a wide range of stress-related disorders including headache, insomnia, indigestion, irritable bowel syndrome and lower backache, to name but a few.

Professional aromatherapy is a safe and appropriate complementary therapy for men and women, children and the elderly, and, in most cases, for those with chronic or serious illnesses such as osteoarthritis, heart disease and cancer. While it is certainly not a replacement for orthodox health care, it does not interfere with medical treatment – and indeed will support the healing process.

■ The above information is from the International Federation of Professional Aromatherapists' web site: www.the-ifpa.org

Herbal medicine

Frequently asked questions

What is herbal medicine?

Herbal medicine is the use of plant remedies in the treatment of disease. It is the oldest known form of medicine.

Our ancestors, by trial and error, found the most effective local plants to heal their illnesses. Now, with the advancement of science enabling us to identify the chemical constituents within these plants, we can better understand their healing powers.

Herbalism, in this country, is now classed as an 'alternative' or 'complementary' discipline but it is still the most widely practised form of medicine worldwide with over 80% of the world's population relying on herbs for health.

The herbalist's approach

Medical herbalists are trained in the same diagnostic skills as orthodox doctors but take a more holistic approach to illness. The underlying cause of the problem is sought and, once identified, it is this which is treated, rather than the symptoms alone. The reason for this is that treatment or suppression of symptoms will not rid the body of the disease itself. Herbalists use their remedies to restore the balance of the body thus enabling it to mobilise its own healing powers.

The first consultation will generally take at least an hour. The herbalist will take notes on the patient's medical history and begin to build a picture of the person as a whole being. Healing is a matter of teamwork with patient, practitioner and the prescribed treatment all working together to restore the body to health.

Treatment may include advice about diet and lifestyle as well as the herbal medicine.

The second appointment may follow in two weeks, subsequent ones occurring monthly – this will depend on the individual herbalist, the patient and the illness concerned.

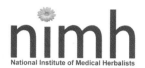

Herbalists use a wide range of plant-based materials for internal and external use. Preparations such as tinctures, fluid extracts, syrups, capsules and creams are all produced to a very high standard.

How do herbs work?

People have always relied on plants for food to nourish and sustain the body. Herbal medicine can be seen in the same way.

Plants with a particular affinity for certain organs or systems of the body are used to 'feed' and restore to health those parts which have become weakened. As the body is strengthened so is its power and ability to fight off disease and when balance and harmony are restored, health will be regained.

What are the differences between herbs and pharmaceutical drugs?

Many of the pharmaceutical drugs used today are based on plant constituents and, even now, when scientists are seeking new 'cures' for disease it is to the plant world that they turn. They find, extract and then synthesise in the laboratory a single active constituent from the plant (the active constituent is the part of the plant that has a therapeutic value), this can then be manufactured on a large scale.

Herbal drugs, however, are extracts from a part of the whole plant (e.g. leaves, roots, berries etc.) and contain hundreds, perhaps thousands of plant constituents.

Herbalists believe that the active constituents are balanced within the plant and are made more (or less) powerful by the numerous other substances present.

For example, the herb *Ephedra sinica* is the source of the alkaloid ephedrine which is used, in orthodox medicine, to treat asthma and nasal congestion but it has the side effect of raising blood pressure.

Within the whole plant are six other alkaloids one of which prevents a rise in blood pressure. Synthetic diuretics (drugs that increase the flow of urine) seriously reduce the potassium level in the body, this has to be restored using potassium supplements. The herbalist uses dandelion leaves which are a potent diuretic but contain potassium to replace naturally that which is lost.

What can herbal medicine treat?

Herbal medicine can treat almost any condition that patients might take to their doctor. Common complaints seen by herbalists include skin problems such as psoriasis, acne and eczema, digestive disorders such as peptic ulcers, colitis, irritable bowel syndrome and indigestion. Problems involving the heart and circulation like angina, high blood pressure, varicose veins, varicose ulcers etc. can also be treated successfully as can gynaecological disorders like premenstrual syndrome and menopausal problems, also conditions such as arthritis, insomnia, stress, migraine and headaches, tonsillitis, influenza and allergic responses like hayfever and asthma.

Herbal medicine offers a safe, gentle and effective approach to health care and serves to promote health as a positive state. It is suitable for all from the very young to the very old.

Qualified herbalists know when a condition is best seen by a doctor or another therapist.

■ The above information is from the National Institute of Medical Herbalists' web site which can be found at www.nimh.org.uk

© *National Institute of Medical Herbalists*

Homeopathy simply explained

Information from the Society of Homeopaths

Starting homeopathic treatment

Homeopathy is an effective and scientific system of healing which assists the natural tendency of the body to heal itself. It recognises that all symptoms of ill health are expressions of disharmony within the whole person and that it is the patient who needs treatment not the disease.

As a new patient, these ideas may be new to you, but homeopathy has been established for about 200 years.

What is homeopathy?

In 1796 a German doctor, Samuel Hahnemann, discovered a different approach to the cure of the sick which he called homeopathy (from the Greek words meaning 'similar suffering'). Like Hippocrates two thousand years earlier he realised that there were two ways of treating ill health, the way of opposites and the way of similars.

Take, for example, a case of insomnia. The way of opposites (conventional medicine or allopathy) is to treat this by giving a drug to bring on an artificial sleep. This frequently involves the use of large or regular doses of drugs which can sometimes cause side effects or addiction.

The way of similars, the homeopathic way, is to give the patient a minute dose of a substance, such as coffee, which in large doses causes sleeplessness in a healthy person. Perhaps surprisingly this will enable the patient to sleep naturally.

Homeopathic remedies cannot cause side effects and you cannot become addicted to them. This is because only a very minute amount of the active ingredient is used in a specially prepared form.

Your homeopath will give you a homeopathic medicine or remedy which matches your symptoms as you

The Society of Homeopaths
representing professional homeopaths

experience them. This also takes account of you as a person – your individual characteristics emotionally as well as physically.

How does it work?

Homeopathic remedies work by stimulating the body's own healing power. This stimulus will assist your own system to clear itself of any expressions of imbalance. The aim is to get you to a level of health so that eventually you will need infrequent treatment.

What will your homeopath need to know?

In order to find the right remedy for you as an individual, your homeopath will need to know all about you. A detailed understanding of who you are, along with any complaints and details of how you experience them, is needed to assess your case correctly. So anything you can tell your homeopath that is typical of who you are will help this process. Finding out about your general energy level, your past medical history and the way you live is also important. Anything you say will be treated in the strictest confidence. The initial consultation may last an hour or more.

What will the treatment be like?

Your homeopath will give you a homeopathic remedy, usually in the

---

Homeopathic remedies work by stimulating the body's own healing power

---

form of a tablet or tablets, occasionally as powders, which should be allowed to dissolve in your mouth; or you may be given a liquid remedy with instructions. Nothing else should be put in the mouth for 20 minutes before or after taking the tablet, not even toothpaste or cigarettes. Your homeopath will usually advise you to avoid coffee, peppermint and preparations containing menthol, eucalyptus and camphor, as these can interfere with the action of the homeopathic remedy. Do make sure that you understand the instructions before you leave.

If you are given homeopathic remedies to take at a later date be sure to store them in a cool dark place, away from anything with a strong smell. If you travel do not let the remedies go through the X-ray.

Please tell your homeopath about any medicine or supplement that has been prescribed for you by your doctor or that you take regularly. Also mention any recent or immediate dental treatment. These may possibly interfere with your homeopathic treatment.

Other treatments may affect your homeopathic treatment, so please do not take any form of medication, including homeopathic remedies, without first asking your homeopath, who may be able to give you some first-aid advice. If you develop a cold, headache, or any symptoms that concern you, please discuss them with your homeopath.

What will happen once treatment starts?

After taking your remedy you may notice some changes. Some patients experience a period of exceptional wellbeing and optimism. Sometimes your symptoms can appear to get worse for a short time. This is a good sign that the remedy is taking effect.

Sometimes a cold, rash or some form of discharge may appear as a 'spring cleaning' effect which means your system is going through a cleaning stage. Similarly, old symptoms can reappear, usually for a short period. These symptoms will pass, and must not be treated as they are a very important part of the healing process. If any response to your treatment concerns you, do contact your homeopath as soon as you can, as it is important to know what happens as treatment progresses. You might also want to make notes of any changes and take them with you to discuss at your next appointment.

How long does treatment take?

This depends very much on what sort of illness you have, as well as the other individual characteristics of your case. So it is not realistic for your homeopath to assess this until it can be seen how you respond to the remedies prescribed over some time. It is possible to say that a slowly developing complaint, or one that has been experienced for some years, will not disappear immediately although there may be a response and some improvement quite soon. Other acute complaints may get better more quickly.

Homeopathy cures from the inside, and often outer symptoms, such as a skin complaint, are the last to clear. Be patient! In the long term it is much better for you to be cured of both the cause of your illness and its symptoms, rather than merely relieving or suppressing the symptoms. Remember that every case is different, and no two patients are alike.

If you wish to discontinue your treatment for any reason, your homeopath will talk things over with you.

Is there any advice about diet and lifestyle?

A homeopath will ask you about your usual diet and lifestyle, and may suggest changes, especially if it seems that this is contributing to your illness. Of course, a good basic diet is necessary for good health, with less sugars, fats, alcohol and refined foods. There is an increasing awareness of the benefits of foods free from

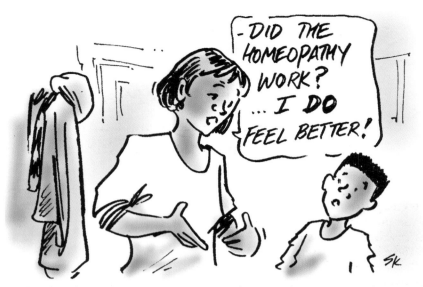

artificial colourings, preservatives and flavourings. Whole foods and organic foods, free from chemical pesticides and fertilisers, are also increasingly available.

What about seeing a GP?

We recommend that you should maintain your relationship with your GP. Your GP will be able to arrange any tests or X-rays you may need. Homeopathy has an alternative philosophy but by working in this way with your GP the two systems of health care can provide complementary services.

It is important that you feel happy with the manner and approach of your homeopath

---

Can I treat myself with homeopathic remedies?

You can use some remedies at home to treat first-aid problems such as cuts, stings, minor burns and bruises. Ask your homeopath for further information or find your nearest class or seminar on this subject.

There are a number of good books available such as:
Homeopathy, Natural Medicine for the Whole Person, by Peter Adams, Element.
Practical Homeopathy, A Complete Guide to Home Treatment, by Beth MacEoin, Bloomsbury.

The Complete Homeopathy Handbook, by Miranda Castro, Macmillan.

How do I find a good homeopath?

To find a good homeopath consult the Register of the Society of Homeopaths. All homeopaths registered with the Society practise in accordance with a Code of Ethics and Practice, hold professional insurance, and have passed stringent academic and clinical assessments before being admitted to the Register.

It is important that you feel happy with the manner and approach of your homeopath. In that way you will be more able to give your homeopath the information needed to prescribe well for you.

Other leaflets available include:
Homeopathy and Foreign Travel, Homeopathy in Pregnancy and Childbirth, Homeopathy, Past Present & Future Medicine, What is Homeopathy?, Homeopathy and the Menopause.

For a copy of these leaflets, or the Society's Register please write, enclosing a stamped, addressed envelope to: The Society of Homeopaths, 11 Brookfield, Duncan Close, Moulton Park, Northampton, NN3 6WL. Tel: 0845 450 6611. Fax: 0845 450 6622 E-mail: info@homeopathy-soh.org Web site: www.homeopathy-soh.org

■ The above information is from the Society of Homeopaths' web site which can be found at www.homeopathy-soh.org

© The Society of Homeopaths

Chinese herbal medicine

Information from the Register of Chinese Herbal Medicine

What is Chinese medicine?

Chinese herbal medicine is one of the great herbal systems of the world, with an unbroken tradition going back to the 3rd century BC. Yet throughout its history it has continually developed in response to changing clinical conditions, and has been sustained by research into every aspect of its use. This process continues today with the development of modern medical diagnostic techniques and knowledge.

Because of its systematic approach and clinical effectiveness it has for centuries had a very great influence on the theory and practice of medicine in the East, and more recently has grown rapidly in popularity in the West. It still forms a major part of healthcare provision in China, and is provided in state hospitals alongside Western medicine.

Chinese medicine includes all oriental traditions emerging from South-east Asia that have their origins in China. Practitioners may work within a tradition that comes from Japan, Vietnam, Taiwan or Korea. It is a complete medical system that is capable of treating a very wide range of conditions. It includes herbal therapy, acupuncture, dietary therapy, and exercises in breathing and movement (tai chi and qi gong). Some or several of these may be employed in the course of treatment

Chinese herbal medicine, along with the other components of Chinese medicine, is based on the concepts of Yin and Yang. It aims to understand and treat the many ways in which the fundamental balance and harmony between the two may be undermined and the ways in which a person's Qi or vitality may be depleted or blocked. Clinical strategies are based upon diagnosis of patterns of signs and symptoms that reflect an imbalance.

However, the tradition as a whole places great emphasis on lifestyle management in order to prevent disease before it occurs. Chinese medicine recognises that health is more than just the absence of disease and it has a unique capacity to maintain and enhance our capacity for wellbeing and happiness.

Herbal medicine and modern pharmacology

There is a growing body of research which indicates that traditional uses of plant remedies and the known pharmacological activity of plant constituents often coincide. However, herbal medicine is distinct from medicine based on pharmaceutical drugs. Firstly, because of the complexity of plant materials it is far more balanced than medicine based on isolated active ingredients and is far less likely to cause side-effects. Secondly, because herbs are typically prescribed in combination, the different components of formulae balance each other, and they undergo a mutual synergy which increases efficacy and enhances safety. Thirdly, herbal medicine seeks primarily to correct internal imbalances rather than to treat symptoms alone, and therapeutic intervention is designed to encourage this self-healing process.

What can Chinese medicine treat?

Chinese medicine is successfully used for a very wide range of conditions. Among the more commonly treated disorders are:

- Skin disease, including eczema, psoriasis, acne, rosacea, urticaria
- Gastro-intestinal disorders, including irritable bowel syndrome, chronic constipation, ulcerative colitis
- Gynaecological conditions, in-

Chinese herbal medicine is one of the great herbal systems of the world

cluding pre-menstrual syndrome and dysmenorrhoea, endometriosis, infertility
- Hepatitis and HIV: some promising results have been obtained for treatment of hepatitis C, and supportive treatment may be beneficial in the case of HIV
- Chronic fatigue syndromes, whether with a background of viral infection or in other situations
- Respiratory conditions, including asthma, bronchitis, and chronic coughs, allergic and perennial rhinitis and sinusitis
- Rheumatological conditions (e.g. osteoarthritis and rheumatoid arthritis)
- Urinary conditions including chronic cystitis
- Psychological problems (e.g. depression, anxiety)
- Children's diseases

Many of these conditions, especially in their chronic forms, create great difficulty for conventional medicine, whilst Chinese herbal medicine has a great deal to offer. The results that can be expected and the length of treatment required will depend on the severity of the condition, its duration, and the general health of the patient.

Who can have treatment?

Chinese medicine can be used by people of any age or constitution. Your practitioner will take any previous or current illness or medication into account before providing treatment. With suitable adjustments for dosage and with some provisos which will be determined by your practitioner, children and pregnant women can very well be treated by Chinese medicine.

What are the herbs like and how much will they cost?

Herbs are now available in a number of formats, both traditional and modern. The traditional method is to boil a mixture of dried herbs to make a tea or to use pills. The herbs are also now commonly prescribed as freeze-dried powders or tinctures. The herbs will at first taste unusual and often bitter to anyone who has not tried them before, but the vast majority of people get used to the taste very quickly.

There are no standard prices for treatment or herbs. This will depend on the individual practitioner and the part of the country you are in. You should enquire about charges when making your appointment. Many private health insurance companies are now covering acupuncture and a few will also pay for herbal treatment. You should contact your insurance company to check.

Are herbs safe?

Chinese herbs are very safe when prescribed correctly by a properly trained practitioner. Over the centuries doctors have compiled detailed information about the pharmacopoeia and placed great emphasis on the protection of the patient. Allergic type reactions are rare, and will cause no lasting damage if treatment is stopped as soon as symptoms appear. All members of

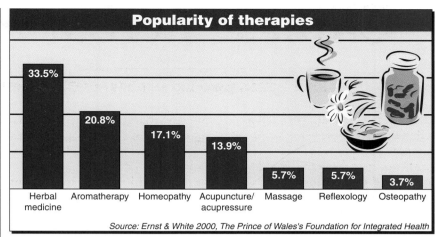

Popularity of therapies

	%
Herbal medicine	33.5%
Aromatherapy	20.8%
Homeopathy	17.1%
Acupuncture/acupressure	13.9%
Massage	5.7%
Reflexology	5.7%
Osteopathy	3.7%

Source: Ernst & White 2000, The Prince of Wales's Foundation for Integrated Health

the RCHM give guidance on this to all patients. The provision of good quality authenticated herbs is also very important to protect public safety, and the RCHM is currently working with the main suppliers and Kew Gardens in order to ensure that the products used by our members meet the highest standards.

Endangered species

The RCHM is greatly concerned about the threats to wild animals and plants that have come as a result of the growth in demand for traditional medicines. We strongly condemn the illegal trade in endangered species and

have a strict policy prohibiting the use of any type of endangered species by any of our Members. The RCHM uses information supplied by the Convention on International Trade in Endangered Species (CITES), the Wildlife Liaison Office of the Metropolitan Police and the Department of the Environment, all of whom work to stop the trade in illegal substances wherever it is found.

■ The above information is from the Register of Chinese Herbal Medicine's web site: www.rchm.co.uk
© The Register of Chinese Herbal Medicine

Reflexology

Information from the Association of Reflexologists

Reflexology is a method of bringing about relaxation, balance and healing through the stimulation of particular points on the feet, or sometimes on the hands. The therapy was known thousands of years ago in China, India and Egypt, but has only recently been practised in the West since it was rediscovered early this century by an American ear, nose and throat surgeon. He noted that pressure on specific parts of the body could have an effect on a related area. Reflex points on the feet and hands are linked to other areas and organs of the body. Tension or congestion in any part of the foot mirrors tension or congestion in a corresponding part, and treating the whole foot can have a deeply relaxing and healing effect on the whole body.

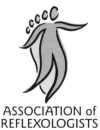

ASSOCIATION of REFLEXOLOGISTS

So how can applying pressure to the feet have an effect elsewhere in the body? Our ancestors walked and ran barefoot over uneven ground. The nerve endings and reflex points on the feet received regular, natural massage as they moved around. Nowadays we spend much of our time sitting down, and when we do walk, it is on hard, flat surfaces, wearing thick-soled shoes to cushion our feet. Women sometimes wear

high heels that alter the balance of pressure on the soles of the feet, putting extra pressure on some areas, and failing to stimulate others. It is very easy for gravity to cause a build-up of waste products and a general stagnation in the feet.

Your body has the ability to heal itself. Correct stimulation of the feet can have a beneficial effect on the whole body. Following illness, stress, injury or disease, it is in a state of 'imbalance', and vital energy pathways are blocked, preventing the body from functioning properly. Reflexology can be used to restore and maintain the body's natural equilibrium and encourage healing.

Reflexologists use their thumbs and fingers to apply gentle pressure to the feet. For each person the application and effect of the therapy is unique. Sensitive, trained hands can detect tiny deposits and imbalances in the feet and by working on these points, the reflexologist can release blockages and restore the free flow of energy to the whole body. Tensions are eased and circulation and elimination are improved. This gentle therapy encourages the body to heal itself at its own pace, often counteracting a lifetime of misuse. This can be an opportunity for you to give time to yourself, time to relax and to replenish your energies.

When you go for a treatment, there will be a preliminary talk with the practitioner. Then you will remove your shoes and socks and relax while the reflexologist begins to work on your feet (or hands if necessary), noting the problem areas. For the most part the treatment is very pleasant and soothing. There may be discomfort in some places but this is fleeting, and is an indication of tension or imbalance in a corresponding part of the body.

Treatment usually lasts for about an hour. A number of sessions will normally be necessary as the benefits of reflexology build up gently and gradually. Weekly treatments are often recommended to begin with, and the total number of sessions will depend on your own body's requirements. Your reflexologist will discuss this with you at the first session. After the first treatment or two, your body may respond in a very definite way: you may have a feeling of wellbeing and relaxation; or you may feel lethargic, nauseous or tearful for a short time. This is transitory and is simply part of the healing process. Once your body is back in tune, it is wise to have regular maintenance treatments.

Our modern lifestyle creates all kinds of physical, emotional and mental stresses. Often we are unable to release these in a natural way and they become 'locked up' in our body, producing a wide range of different symptoms. It has been estimated that more than 75% of all illness is stress-related. Stress can lead to a weakening of our body's defence system so we become more vulnerable to illness and disease. When we are stressed we are tense. Tense muscles restrict the blood flow, reduce the transportation of oxygen and nutrients to all the cells of the body and prevent the proper disposal of waste products. The whole system becomes sluggish and is unable to function efficiently. We may get muscle aches and pains, or we may develop problems in underlying organs. By helping to relax the muscles, by encouraging the process of circulation and the elimination of toxins, and by stimulating the production of natural chemicals in the brain, reflexology can ease pain and discomfort. As tension and irritation are soothed away, and as you become calmer, you will find improvements occurring in many different areas of your life: relationships become more rewarding; you are able to handle work or study more effectively; you sleep better, throw off fatigue more easily, gain mental alertness and generally enjoy life more.

Recent research suggests that reflexology can help reduce sick leave by 25% or more

Recent research suggests that reflexology can help reduce sick leave by 25% or more. Some firms are now beginning to introduce this therapy as a service to their employees, helping to maintain their optimum health and well-being.

The benefits of reflexology can be enjoyed by anyone: a young baby having sleeping trouble; a 90-year-old looking for relief from the aches and pains of old age; the mother looking for a break from the demands of her family; those coping with the pressures of work or unemployment;

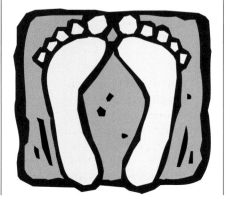

the sports enthusiast looking for balancing and conditioning and speedy recovery from soreness and injury; the teenager coping with the hormonal see-saw of a growing body; people in sedentary occupations; people on their feet all day. Reflexology stimulates energy flow, and helps to produce a glowing skin and bright eyes, a clear mind, a renewed capacity for enjoyment, the appearance and feeling of positive well-being. Reflexology can enhance your everyday life, keeping you at your peak. Regular preventative treatments help to strengthen the body and ward off illness and fatigue. An increasing number of people are using this safe, natural therapy as a way of relaxing, balancing and harmonising the body.

When choosing a reflexologist, it is wise to ensure that the practitioner has been properly trained at a reputable school or training establishment, works to a professional code of ethics and is fully insured to practise on members of the public. The Association of Reflexologists publishes a Register of qualified practitioners to which the public can refer with confidence.

Should you wish to train as a reflexologist, there are no maximum age limits, although many schools do have a minimum age limit of 18 years. It is probably fair to say that often an older person with more experience of life can bring an additional dimension to the treatment, as the lending of a wise and understanding ear can be most valuable in helping a client to release personal stress and tension.

Reflexology is a practical skill rather than an academic subject, so high academic ability is not necessary. However, courses do include the study of anatomy, physiology and integrated biology, so some facility in this area is essential. It is more important, however, that students should have genuine sensitivity and caring for others and good listening skills. Courses are usually part-time, often at weekends, with study spread over a minimum of nine months and involving a good deal of home study and practical work.

The majority of reflexologists are self-employed and work either from home or from a room rented in a natural health centre or multi-therapy clinic, and some practitioners are prepared to visit their clients' homes to give a treatment. A number of reflexologists give their time in a voluntary capacity to help in hospices, hospitals or homes for the elderly, while others work on a private basis within NHS clinics and Health Centres. It is now possible for fundholding GPs to employ reflexologists on their staff, and non-fundholding GPs may also employ complementary therapists subject to the approval of the Family Health Services Authority. As reflexology works so well with other forms of treatment many doctors are finding that referring patients to reflexo-

> *There is a growing interest in reflexology amongst nurses and health care workers with many undertaking training for use in their own sphere*

logists actually saves them money. There is also a growing interest in reflexology amongst nurses and health care workers with many undertaking training for use in their own sphere.

This information has been prepared by the Association of Reflexologists. The Association is an independent organisation, founded in 1984 with the aim of setting standards for reflexology and providing a network of qualified and experienced practitioners. Full members of the Association use the designated letters MAR after their names, and are included on the Register of Practitioners.

For all reflexology information and to find a reflexologist contact the Association of Reflexologists, 27 Old Gloucester Street, London, WC1N 3XX. Tel: 0870 567 3320. Fax: 01823 336646. E-mail: info@aor.org.uk Web site: www.aor.org.uk

Iridology

Information from the Guild of Naturopathic Iridologists

Introduction

Iridology complements all therapeutic sciences because it provides vital information needed in order to establish the root cause of ailments, revealing the appropriate treatments required.

Iridology is a safe, non-invasive diagnostic science, which can be integrated with both orthodox and complementary medicine.

Iridology helps the patient learn about their strengths and weaknesses and become more aware of what they can do to help themselves. The iridologist will guide the patient as to the best ways of reversing existing conditions and managing genetic weaknesses.

What is it?

Iridology is the study of the 'iris' of the eye – the exposed nerve endings which make up the coloured part of the eye, each of which are connected to the brain.

A trained iridologist sees the exposed nerve endings as a 'map', revealing information about:
- the body's genetic strengths and weaknesses,
- levels of inflammation and toxaemia,

- the efficiency of the eliminative systems and organs.

In the hands of those who are well versed in the pathology of the pathways of disease, as well as anatomy and physiology, this provides a veritable microchip of information.

History

In the 17th, 18th and 19th centuries, writings and works on iris markings and their meanings were recorded, mainly by medical practitioners.

One of the earliest was Dr Ignatz von Peczely, a Hungarian doctor. While still a child he accidentally broke the leg of an owl. He noticed a black mark appearing in the owl's eye, which over time changed in form and shading.

Ignatz von Peczely qualified in medicine at the Vienna Medical College in 1867. He had ample opportunity to study the irides of patients before and after surgery,

systematically recording, correlating and publishing his research in the book *Discoveries in the Realms of Nature and Art of Healing*. His *Iris Chart* was established in 1880.

In the 1860s, a young Swedish boy, Nils Liljequist, became ill as the consequence of a vaccination, followed by doses of quinine and iodine. He noticed the changes in colour of his formerly blue eyes, as the drug spots appeared.

In 1870, he published a paper describing his experiences, *Quinine and Iodine change the Colour of the Iris*, and in 1893 published *Om Oegendiagnosen*, which included his 'Iris Chart'.

We should not be surprised that Liljequist and von Peczely's 'Iris Charts' were very similar.

About iris constitutions

The 3 main constitutional types
There are 3 main iris colour types, namely brown, blue and grey. There is also an exception to these basic types known as a Biliary or Mixed Constitution, namely part blue and part brown. This type displays a combination of factors that are found in both the blue- and the brown-eyed types.

Where the iris pigmentation is slight, the iris appears blue as is commonly found in the northern European type, where less pigmentation is required for protection against intense sunlight. On the other hand, with an increase in pigmentation, the colour becomes more grey and proceeds to brown and on to dark brown, as is found in the Mediterranean, Middle Eastern, African and Indian types. Over the generations, interbreeding has, in some instances, produced a mixed genotype known as a Biliary Constitution, where the person inherits the strengths and weaknesses of both the brown- and blue-eyed constitutions.

We are therefore left with 3 distinct groupings:
- the blue-eyed constitution known as the Lymphatic Type;
- the pure brown-eyed constitution known as the Haematogenic Type;
- and the combination of the two being the Mixed or Biliary Type.

The Lymphatic constitutional type
The lymphatic constitution is considered a Lymphatic Type due to an overproliferation of lymphatic cells which respond to irritations, inflammations and a build-up of excess mucous and catarrh. This in turn means that this type is more likely to encounter inflammatory conditions of the joints, allergies, respiratory and skin disorders.
- Constitution – Lymphatic
- Type – Pure Lymphatic
- Iris Colour – Blue
- Description – Loose wavy fibres, like combed hair in a blue or grey iris.
- Inherent Tendencies – Reactivity of the lymphatic system (adenoid and tonsil irritations; splenitis; swollen lymph nodes; irritated appendix; catarrh with exudations; eczema; acne; flakey, dry skin; dandruff; asthma; coughs; bronchitis; sinusitis; diarrhoea; arthritis; vaginal discharge; eye irritations; fluid retention).

The Haematogenic constitutional type
The true brown eye reflects the

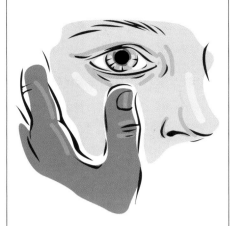

haematogenic constitution which is more prone to gastro-intestinal, liver, pancreatic, endocrine and blood disturbances.
- Constitution – Haematogenic
- Iris Colour – Brown to Deep Brown
- Description – A true brown iris, with no underlying colours. The texture resembles velvet with few features. Under microscopic examination, however, fine differentiations are apparent. There are numerous chromatophorous cells and the stroma is therefore difficult to distinguish, with markings located mainly in the sectorial zone. Occasional lighter zones are present which give the appearance of sandpaper and indicate areas of inflammation or irritation. These are sometimes found in the heart and/or kidney zones and can be indicative of organic disease in these organs. Cramp rings and radials are often present as are anaemia, sodium or cholesterol rings.

It is not uncommon with this particular constitutional type to find brown blemishes on the sciera indicating latent hepatitis.

(The Oriental haematogenic is usually of a light yellow brown, with a texture resembling rough sandpaper when viewed under a microscope.)
- Inherent Tendencies – Anaemia; lack of catalysts (iron, gold, arsenic, copper, zinc, iodine); blood diseases (hepatitis, jaundice); muscle spasms; arthritis; chronic degenerative illness; endocrine disorders (thyroid, adrenals and pituitary); spleenic

disturbances; poor lymphatic drainage; swollen glands; Hodgkin's Disease; flatulance; constipation; colonic tumour; dyspepsia; digestive disorders with lowered enzymatic production; frequent intolerance to cow's milk; ulcers; liver, gall-bladder and pancreatic malfunctions; diabetes; circulatory disorders; auto-intoxication.

The Biliary constitutional type
The mixed or biliary constitution, whilst being prone to disturbances exhibited by both the Lymphatic and Haematogenic Types, is, in the main, more prone to liver, gall bladder and pancreatic disturbances, flatulence, constipation, diabetes and blood diseases.
- Constitution – Biliary
- Iris Colour – Basic Blue background with a brown overlay. The iris often appears light brown to greenish brown; sometimes described as the hazel eye.
- Description – In many cases the iris appears uniformly brown and is therefore often confused with the Haematogenic Constitution. Deeper observation however reveals that only the upper, cryptic leaf shows brown pigmentation with the lower leaf showing through as bluey-green. Usually, however, the iris will show clear areas of blue and contrasting brown areas. Contraction rings are often in evidence as is the darkened central area (central heterochromia). Sometimes sectorial heterochromia is evident. Occasionally, lymphatic tophi of various hues are also present.
- Inherent Tendencies – Flatulence; constipation; colitis; hypoglycaemia; diabetes; blood diseases; gall-stones; liver, gall-bladder, bile duct and pancreatic disorders; gastro-intestinal weakness with spasm; Haematogenic and Lymphatic Constitutional strengths and weaknesses.

- The above information is from the Guild of Naturopathic Iridologists' web site which can be found at www.gni-international.org

Naturopathy definitions

Information from the General Council and Register of Naturopaths

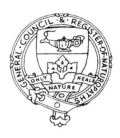

What is naturopathy or naturopathic medicine?

Naturopathic medicine is the field of health care which works with the body's own efforts to allow optimum expression of physiological, mental/emotional, and physical health, given the individual's genetic make-up and environment.

Naturopathy is an approach to health care that promotes and maintains health. It recognises that there are laws governing human function and our natural environment:

■ Every living thing has a vitality, this is known as the principle of vitalism.

■ There is a healing power in nature. The body heals itself because of its innate vitality. A medicine given to a cadaver will produce no effects; thus medicines act only to stimulate the innate healing power of the body.

■ There is an invariable connection between the structural, biochemical and mental/emotional elements of all living beings. This is known as the triad of health.

■ There is an interaction of the whole person; dysfunction in one part of the body inevitably leads to dysfunction elsewhere, just as dysfunction in one part of the naturopathic triad means all parts of the triad will be affected.

■ People are genetically, biochemically, structurally and emotionally different from one another: they are individuals.

■ We interact with our environment; health is a reflection of a harmonious interaction.

■ There is an important difference between acute and chronic disease. Acute diseases are the result of the expression of the body's homoeostatic mechanisms attempting to re-establish balance. For example a high fever is produced to combat infection in order to aid the immunological defence mechanisms.

■ All disease starts with a disruption to the body's homoeostatic mechanisms; health is a return to balance of these mechanisms.

■ Health is more than the absence of disease; health is when all aspects of an individual's biochemical, mental/emotional and physical being are in balance.

■ The human body has adapted to its environment over millions of years, it has come to expect certain foods for its fuel, clean water, a certain amount of fresh air and sunlight, and a certain amount of exercise and rest/relaxation.

Naturopathic medicine is the application of these laws in a clinical setting to maintain, improve or establish health in patients. It is therefore not a technique but an approach to health care.

The defining elements of naturopathy are:

1. That it always seeks to work with the body's own self-correcting mechanisms, or efforts to maintain homoeostasis.

2. That it always attempts to address all three aspects of the naturopathic triad.

3. That it regards education of the patient as highly as treatment of the patient.

4. That it always seeks to address lifestyle factors that are contributing to the problem and re-educate the patient into a lifestyle more conducive to health.

■ The above information is from the General Council and Register of Naturopaths' web site: www.naturopathy.org.uk

© General Council and Register of Naturopaths

> *Naturopathic medicine is the field of health care which works with the body's own efforts to allow optimum expression of physiological, mental/emotional, and physical health*

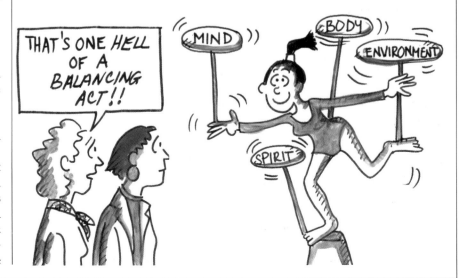

What is spiritual healing and what does it do?

Information from the National Federation of Spiritual Healers (NFSH)

Spiritual healing is a completely natural process that helps us achieve better health and a sense of well-being. This is brought about by transmitting healing energies through the person giving the healing to the person receiving the healing. It could be described as kick-starting the natural resources of the person receiving healing (the patient) and giving a boost to energy levels, but at the same time it relaxes the patient so that he or she can deal with illness or injury in the best possible way. It can be helpful, sometimes to a remarkable degree, to all kinds of conditions, not just physical illness, but psychological, spiritual and emotional problems too. Indeed, the medically diagnosed nature of the illness appears to be irrelevant to the outcome and case histories bear witness to the important contribution healing can make whatever prompts a person to seek healing.

Spiritual healing is a completely natural process that helps us achieve better health and a sense of well-being

In addition to its value in relieving pain and restoring function, healing is also notable for initiating improvements in patients' attitudes and quality of life.

There are various healing organisations in the United Kingdom and the National Federation of Spiritual Healers (NFSH), which was founded in 1954, is generally acknowledged to be the principal organisation with more than 5,500 members working individually and in Healing Centres throughout the country. The NFSH and some other healing organisations are not associated with any particular religion, -ism or -ology. They see the source of healing as divine, but respect the right of every individual to his or her own interpretation of that source. The word 'spiritual' in the title refers to that quality of spirituality implicit in the healing process. In recent years a new group called UK Healers has been established by several healing organisations collaborating for the public good. UK Healers is working towards voluntary self-regulation for healers and the number of organisations involved has grown steadily.

Healers work in their own and patients' homes, in the workplace, in doctors' surgeries, hospitals, healing centres, therapy rooms and many other situations. When you attend a healing session you should find it informal and relaxing. Some people are worried that they may be asked to remove their clothing – this should not happen – although of course you may be more comfortable removing a coat or shoes. All healers have their own way of working but usually you sit on a chair or stool, or you may be asked to lie down on a treatment couch, and the healer generally works with his or her hands a short distance from your body and only touches you after first asking your consent, and then very gently and appropriately (i.e. no touching of areas that could cause offence). All NFSH healers have attended training courses, have experienced self-development and are bound by a Code of Conduct.

You may feel a variety of sensations as the healing goes to work. Warmth, coolness, pressure, tingling, pain coming then going, all these are signals that something is happening, but even if you feel very little this does not mean that the process is not working. Healing seeks out the underlying cause as well as the 'presenting' symptom and is often about restoring balance to your life, about feelings and relationships with others. It may even prompt changes in lifestyle to help you regain control of your life and bring about a sense of proportion and feeling that your feet are firmly on the ground. There are no harmful side effects and spiritual healing works well with any other therapy. It works alongside any treatment the doctor may be giving and it is a process, above all, to help you to help yourself.

It can be helpful to all kinds of conditions, not just physical illness, but psychological, spiritual and emotional problems too

Sometimes spiritual healing is referred to as faith healing. To benefit from healing you do not need faith. Nothing special is expected except perhaps an open mind and a degree of trust in the healer.

■ If you want to know more or contact a healer in your area, the National Federation of Spiritual Healers (NFSH) offers information and a referral service. People who want to become healers with NFSH need to be 18 years of age or over and NFSH welcomes all enquiries. The number to contact is 0845 123 2767 (local call rate line) and NFSH telephone lines are open from 10 am to 4 pm weekdays. See page 41 for full contact details.

© National Federation of Spiritual Healers (NFSH)

GPs offer patients complementary medicine

Half of general practices offer patients complementary medicine

By Roger Dobson,
Abergavenny

Half of general practices in England now offer patients some access to complementary or alternative medicines.

New research shows that there has been a substantial increase in provision since 1995, when a similar study by the same authors found that 40% of practices were offering complementary or alternative medicines.

'Increased provision by the primary health care team, coupled with its use for priority patient groups, suggests that CAM [complementary or alternative medicine] is regarded by many GPs as having a role to play in patient management,' says a report of the study in *Family Practice* (2003:20:575-7). The growth in services has been made possible partly by asking patients to pay for the services, the report says.

In the study, a postal questionnaire was sent to one in eight GP partnerships in England, and 870 took part. The survey in 1995, which also sampled one in eight partnerships, had found that 40% were offering access to complementary or alternative medicines, and the authors, from the Medical Care Research Unit, at the University of Sheffield, wanted to see if there had been any changes.

They estimate that almost half the general practices in England (49%) were providing some access to complementary or alternative therapies in 2001. One or more members of the primary healthcare team – GPs, nurses, and others – provided the therapies in an estimated 30% of practices; independent practitioners worked in 12% of practices; and 27% of practices made NHS referrals to external providers.

The proportion of practices offering therapies and whose primary healthcare team provides the therapies had increased by 38% since 1995,

and acupuncture and homeopathy are the therapies most frequently provided in this way, says the report. Involvement of an independent practitioner working at the practice has doubled since 1995, and these practitioners most often provide manipulative therapies. The percentage of practices making NHS referrals for complementary or alternative therapies has changed little. The proportion of services supported by full or partial payments by patients rose from 26% to 42% between 1995 and 2001.

In 2001, complementary or alternative therapies were being used

---

The proportion of services supported by full or partial payments by patients rose from 26% to 42% between 1995 and 2001

---

to provide support or care for each of the NHS priority groups. Eleven per cent of practices used the therapies for cancer patients; 10% for elderly patients; 9% for mental health patients; and 5% each for patients with diabetes or coronary heart disease.

The report says that the increase in the proportion of practices with an independent practitioner in complementary or alternative medicine is surprising, given the known difficulties in sustaining funding for such services: 'This growth appears to have been facilitated in part by requesting patient payments. Assuming that these services are provided according to perceived patient need, the reported growth in patient payment for these services has clear equity implications.'

It adds, 'To meet acceptable standards of clinical governance, more evidence is needed regarding the CAM qualifications and training of all those providing this type of care to NHS primary care patients.'

■ The above information is from the *British Medical Journal*, 2003; 327:1250 with permission from the BMJ Publishing Group.

© 2004 BMJ Publishing Group

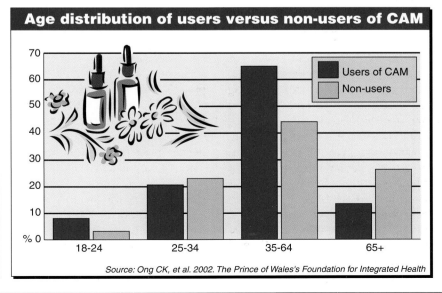

Age distribution of users versus non-users of CAM

Source: Ong CK, et al. 2002. The Prince of Wales's Foundation for Integrated Health

When there's no real alternative

One in five of us regularly uses complementary medicine, but how much of it really works, and when does it become dangerous? Lucy Atkins reports

When Stephen Hall, 43, was diagnosed with inoperable pancreatic cancer, he did what many of us might and went to an alternative therapist who promised him that his condition was curable. Hall believed him. Last week, his 'wellness practitioner', Reginald Gill, 68, from Poole, Dorset, was convicted of two offences under the Trades Descriptions Act after selling Hall an 'IFAS high frequency therapy device' that would, he claimed, kill off the cancer cells. Gill had also advised Hall against chemotherapy, saying he would 'go home in a box' if he did, and told him to stop taking morphine for the pain.

Instead, he put him on an extreme diet, sold him an electronic device, and charged him £75 for treatment sessions at home. The court heard that Gill told Hall after one treatment: 'I've got it. I've killed the bad cells; it's just the pancreas that needs more work.'

Hall died 10 weeks after the cancer was diagnosed. Last week, his mother said outside the court: 'The verdict today should go a long way towards protecting the sick and the terminally ill who, in good faith, go to bogus practitioners who make false claims . . . Stephen was a hostage to the treatment that the so-called clinic advocated, so depriving him of any sense of normality in the last weeks of his life.' Gill will be sentenced in January.

Clearly, the promises of complementary and alternative medicines (Cams) can be immensely seductive. About one in five of us uses them regularly and millions swear that some therapies cure anything from stress to cancer. But when good sense is replaced by blind faith and a mistrust in conventional medicine, the use of Cams can backfire.

Last year in Melbourne, Australia, Isabella Denley, an epileptic toddler, died after her parents ditched the anti-convulsant medication she had been prescribed by her neurologist. The drugs had terrible side effects, including sleep loss and hyperactivity, so they turned to alternative therapies, visiting a vibrational kinesiologist, a cranial osteopath and a psychic who told them Isabella was suffering from a past-life trauma.

Finding out which therapies work for which conditions can be confusing

---

An inquest heard that when she died, the toddler was exclusively on homeopathic medication. Her parents believed they were doing their utmost. But clearly the potential pitfalls of Cams go beyond ruthless charlatans. Indeed, the real peril may be our faith that alternative therapies will inevitably reach – and cure – the parts that allopathic medicines will not.

'There is certainly evidence to show that some therapies are effective for certain conditions,' says a spokesperson for the Research Council for Complementary Medicine (RCCM). But finding out which ones work for which conditions can be confusing. Often several studies of the same therapy will contradict each other, and since funding for research is hard to come by many studies are considered flawed.

The RCCM has a database with about 85,000 citations of clinical trials and research outcomes and has just received government funding to assess the quality and outcome of twelve therapies in the four NHS priority areas – cancer, coronary heart disease, mental health and chronic conditions. But so far, few Cams have been clinically proven to work.

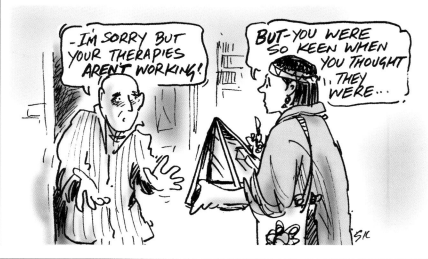

Indeed, hardly a week goes by when a study doesn't appear to disprove some Cam or other. In December 2003, one in the *British Medical Journal* showed that evening primrose oil – until recently available on the NHS to treat eczema – doesn't help the condition after all. Also in December 2003 the University of Washington in Seattle published findings that echinacea is no better than a placebo when it comes to treating colds in children.

Naturally, such scientific scepticism does not stop millions of us from using Cams. A recent report by Virgin money found that 'spiritual spending' has soared in Britain to £670m a year (on yoga, acupuncture, massage and other such therapies). And, according to the Prince of Wales's Foundation for Integrated Health (FIH), about 20% of British people use one of eight alternative therapies (acupuncture, aroma-therapy, chiropractic, homeopathy, hypnotherapy, medical herbalism, osteopathy and reflexology) between 2.8 to 5.3 times a year.

Many people use alternative remedies successfully for minor ailments and overall wellness. Others however turn to Cams in desperation after a devastating diagnosis, believing they have nothing to lose. Around 75% of breast cancer patients are estimated to have tried alter-native therapies and many cancer specialists believe Cams do have an important role in pain management. Sarah Parkinson, wife of comedian Paul Merton, who died this year of breast cancer, turned in her last months to alternative therapies instead of chemotherapy, having decided that, for her, quality of life was paramount. But other cancer patients switch to alternative remedies believing they will be saved.

Doctors warn of the dangers of 'pseudo-scientific' cancer remedies, such as shark's cartilage and mistletoe, which are put forward as miracle cancer cures. These, they say, are causing some patients who may benefit from conventional medicine to ditch it entirely, sometimes with dire consequences. One study this year in the *European Journal of Cancer* found that the death rate for cancer patients who were also users of alternative medicine was greater than for non-users. While no conclusions were reached about why this was, some doctors believe it is a misplaced faith that may lead us to eschew conventional treatments, such as chemotherapy, that could save our lives.

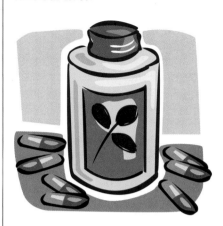

So, do we put too much faith in alternative therapies? Many of us, when we get some new symptom, now turn to a trusted alternative therapist without first seeing our GP. Of course, most reputable therapists will immediately refer you to a doctor if your symptoms seem worrying. But what if they don't? Misdiagnosis – or failure entirely to diagnose a serious condition – can have devastating consequences. James Turner, an 11-year-old Canadian boy, was taken to a chiropractor by his parents when he developed chest pains while swimming in July 2000. The chiro-practor twice adjusted his neck and back without taking X-rays. Soon after, James was rushed to a children's hospital, having lost control of his legs and bowels. He was given an MRI and neurosurgery for a benign tumour (a ganglioglioma) on his spinal cord.

This type of tumour is non-cancerous and slow-growing – with proper detection and medical treat-ment about 75% of afflicted children escape paralysis if the spinal cord is undamaged at the time of diagnosis. James's tumour, however, had been damaged (the parents, who are suing the chiropractor, say this was caused by the chiropractor's manipulation). James is now a paraplegic.

Nobody is saying that chiro-practic *per se* is dangerous (indeed, many studies show it can be very beneficial for certain conditions). Chiropractors, and therapists from other established disciplines such as osteopathy or homeopathy state openly that they are not (necessarily) trained physicians. But still we assume they will spot any danger signs. Dr Stephen Zeitzew, chief of orthopaedic surgery at the West Los Angeles Veterans Administration Healthcare Centre, speaks for many doctors when he says this is a tall order: 'Often diagnosis and treatment is challenging even to physicians with particular expertise. It is clearly true that on occasion the lack of diagnosis [by Cam practitioners] puts our patients in danger'.

Such concerns echo a seminal House of Lords report in 2000 which warned: 'One of the main dangers of Cam is that patients could miss out on conventional medical diagnosis and treatment because they choose only to consult a Cam practitioner.' Zeitzew also points out that if your chosen practitioner is less than above board, the risks accelerate.

One alternative 'helpline' was recently singled out by *Which?* magazine for giving misleading advice on prostate problems after a doctor phoned, posing as a concerned member of the public and describing symptoms of prostate cancer. The doctor was offered an expensive herbal supplement and told that his symptoms were not necessarily anything to worry about.

Of the eight most popular therapies in Britain, only two (chiropractic and osteopathy) are regulated by law in the same way dentists, doctors and nurses are. Acupuncture and herbal practi-tioners could be about to follow suit. 'Things are changing,' says Simon Mills, research coordinator of the University of Exeter's comple-mentary health programme. 'Practi-tioners are recognising their respons-ibility to the public, to patients, and to themselves.'

But most currently rely on self-regulation by organisational bodies to ensure high standards, safety and accountability. 'Choose an alter-native therapist who belongs to a reputable professional body,' advises Mills. If you go to a herbalist it is particularly important that the herbs come from reputable sources (the National Institute of Medical Herbalists and the Register of Traditional Chinese Medicine provide fully trained practitioners).

Michael MacIntyre, chairman of the European Herbal Practitioners Association (www.euroherb.com) says: 'You should always ask whether they belong to a credible organisation with a code of practice and disciplinary procedure, and whether they have insurance.'

The Foundation for Integrated Health is also about to publish guidelines on how to choose a practitioner, and anyone considering alternative therapy would be wise to consult them. The bottom line is clear: the vast majority of alternative therapists are well trained and reputable.

Cams themselves are rarely dangerous. But the way we use them just might be.

So do they work?

Herbal medicine

Use of plant extracts to treat wide variety of disorders and maintain good health – physically and mentally. About 30% of the population spends about £31m a year on herbal remedies.

Does it work?

Professor Edzard Ernst, Britain's only professor of complementary medicine, wrote in the *British Medical Journal* this October: 'The evidence on herbal medicines is incomplete, complex, and confusing.' A recent overview of herbal medicine included 23 systematic reviews of rigorous trials of herbal medicines. Eleven came to a positive conclusion, nine yielded promising but not convincing results, and three were negative.

Dangers

Between 1968 and 1997, the World Health Organization's monitoring centre collected 8,985 reports of adverse incidents associated with herbal medicines from 55 countries. Ernst points out that this number amounts to only a tiny fraction of adverse events associated with conventional drugs held in the same database.

'Choose an alternative therapist who belongs to a reputable professional body'

Risks

Unreliable sources, adulteration of Chinese herbal treatments with synthetic drugs, misbranding, lack of standardisation, possible side effects (one study found that some herbs, such as St John's wort, gingko biloba and echinacea in high doses could reduce fertility). Also a possible danger of reactions with prescription drugs.

Some banned herbs

Aristolochi: for 'nephrotoxicity' (kidney damage). Kava: for causing 'heptatoxicity' (liver damage). Ephedra: banned in the US by the International Olympic Committee, the National Football League, the National Collegiate Athletic Association, minor league baseball, and the US armed forces following some deaths from overuse.

Chiropractic

Treats musculo-skeletal complaints by adjusting muscles, tendons and joints using manipulation and massage techniques (as does osteopathy, said to have similar benefits to chiropractic).

Does it work?

The 2000 House of Lords report states

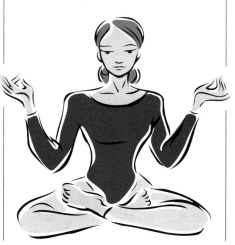

that there is 'good evidence of the efficacy of osteopathy and chiropractic. Indeed, they appear to be somewhat more effective than the manipulative techniques employed by conventional physiotherapists.'

Dangers

Misdiagnosis or failure to diagnose specific conditions. See a GP for a diagnosis and/or referral.

Homeopathy

Treats a wide range of physical and mental complaints using minute dilutions of animal, vegetable and mineral substances that in higher doses could be harmful. This is said to stimulate the body to heal itself. According to the WHO, homeopathy is the second most commonly used form of health care in the world after herbal medicine.

Does it work?

Huge, ongoing scientific debate. Homeopathic solutions are diluted so many times that many scientists argue they are unlikely to contain any of the original ingredients at all. But in 2001 a study found that dissolved molecules do not simply spread out in a regular fashion in the solution but tend to clump together in bigger clusters of molecules – and then as even bigger lumps composed of these clusters. This could explain how a heavily diluted homeopathic remedy might contain more of the 'active' ingredient than expected.

Individual remedies produce varied scientific results: one hayfever trial found a noticeable improvement in patients taking a homeopathic remedy over those in the control group. Another recent trial found that arnica does nothing to reduce pain or accelerate healing after surgery.

Dangers

Misdiagnosis/failure to diagnose serious conditions.

Acupuncture

The House of Lords report said: 'There is also scientific evidence of the efficacy of acupuncture, notably for pain relief and the treatment of nausea.'

© *Guardian Newspapers Limited 2003*

The alternative professor

Sarah Boseley meets the world-class scientist who turned his back on the Viennese medical elite to become the UK's first (and only) professor of complementary medicine

Just over a decade ago, Edzard Ernst's name would have been whispered with deference in the corridors of one of the most prestigious medical schools in the world. He held the chair of physical and rehabilitation medicine at the Medical Faculty of Vienna, a city where medicine has huge status and practitioners such as Sigmund Freud waltzed into legend. Ernst presided over the biggest department of its kind in Europe, with 120 people under him.

But then Ernst did something quite unexpected: he chose to turn his back on all that and head down the path of what some of his peers consider superstition and folklore. 'It was a very big job,' he says of Vienna, smiling. 'A life job. It had all the security and pension and boredom that goes with it.' He quotes a proverb from his native Germany: 'They say when a donkey gets bored, he goes on the ice.'

Ernst launched himself at the thinnest ice one could imagine. This world-class scientist became the first and only professor of complementary medicine in the UK, based in what looks like a large detached house in Exeter. 'I had 3,000 sq metres and 10 secretaries. When I came here I had nothing but havoc,' he says.

Not just havoc but suspicion and downright hostility. Complementary and alternative medicine (CAM) practitioners had been delighted when the building magnate Maurice Laing decided to plough £1.5m into establishing the chair. They were appalled when the post was given to a conventional scientist who declared his intention was to put therapies and treatments from acupuncture to herbs to reflexology under rigorous scrutiny, to find out what worked and what did not. Most CAM practitioners insist that centuries of use are sufficient demonstration that therapies work. Others blame science for most of the world's evils.

> **'At the beginning I had more opposition from mainstream medicine locally. At the hospital and the Trust, they felt they did not need a witch doctor in the first place'**

Ernst admits his one big mistake was not to have understood quite what he was walking into: 'Ten years ago I didn't fully comprehend the situation. On the continent, CAM practitioners would normally be doctors. I didn't realise that there are between 20,000 and 40,000 CAM practitioners in the UK and that most of them would be opposed to what I was planning to do.'

He was caught between a rock and a hard place, because the medical establishment was not keen either and several universities had turned Laing's offer down ('it was hotter than cigarette money').

'At the beginning I had more opposition from mainstream medicine locally. At the hospital and the Trust [in Exeter], they felt they did not need a witch doctor in the first place and certainly not a German witch doctor. A lot of people thought once they had seen what I was up to that it was a waste of talent and money.'

He won most of the mainstream critics over, but failed so regularly with the CAM lobby that after a few years of assiduously attending meetings, giving lectures and trying to convince them of the value of rigorous randomised controlled trials, he gave up: 'They say you can't squeeze a holistic, individualised approach like homeopathy or spiritual healing into the straitjacket

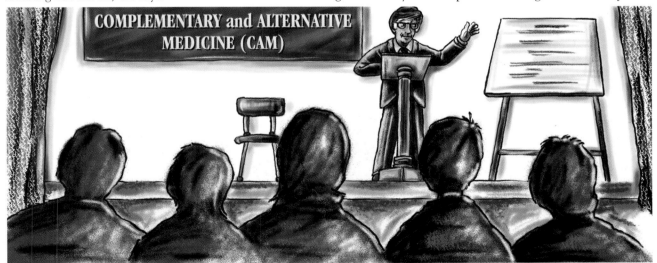

of randomised controlled trials – not that it is the only research tool, but it is a good one. The argument surfaces on a daily basis. It is as frequent as it is wrong.'

For the past few years, he says, he has kept his head down. 'That was successful – anybody can successfully ignore anybody else,' he says ruefully. 'It was also successful in that we produced an awful lot of work and got this unit on the map and we are proud of our achievement. Maybe it is time to re-engage in the dialogue from the powerful position of being the leading centre in the world.'

Ernst has 700 papers published in reputable scientific journals now and a worldwide reputation. 'I know what I'm talking about, whereas 10 years ago, to be frank, it was more of a hobby-horse.'

It is hard to imagine a member of the UK's medical elite devoting their life to complementary medicine. Ernst, however, comes from a culture where alternative therapies have long blended with the mainstream. He is from four generations of conventional doctors but, he says, 'Even as a young boy I was treated with complementary therapies – mostly homeopathy.'

His first post was in a homeopathic hospital in Munich, where he was greatly impressed. 'If you study medicine and pharmacology, you know [homeopathy] can't work,' he says. The active substances in homeopathic medicines are so diluted that pharmacology says they cannot have an effect. 'Then you start working in a homeopathic hospital and people get better. Is that a miracle? It certainly is very impressive for a young doctor.

'Looking back, I wonder if a lot was a placebo effect.' Placebo to him, however, is not a negative. He would never assume people who get better on placebos were not ill in the first place. 'I would like to have an institute of placebo research, but the funding would be even worse. You would get placebo money! But it's absolutely fascinating what's happening there. It is what gels mainstream and complementary medicine together. As doctors, we don't want to realise it. We pride ourselves that therapy does the trick.'

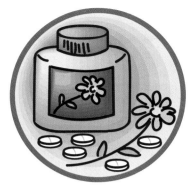

This is a scientist willing to explore the unthinkable and unwilling to be told what to think. Scientific logic says homeopathy cannot work, but Ernst continues to study its therapies not to shoot it down, but in the hope of discovering what it is that does work. He treats his French wife with homeopathy, he says. 'We were both brought up with it.'

But he adds: 'People mistakenly think I must be a promoter of complementary medicine – that I should have an allegiance to the camp. I don't. My allegiance is firstly to the patient – I feel that very strongly as an ex-clinician – and secondly to science. If in the course of that I have to hurt the feelings of homeopaths I regret that, but I can't help it.'

He left Vienna, he says, because medicine there was about power and money and status. 'The Viennese got on my nerves . . . The time they spent intriguing against each other in the faculty could have been spent more fruitfully.' Secondly, he didn't like being an academic administrator when his real love was research. Thirdly, 'I had been in England before as a young doctor in St George's, Tooting, and I always felt this had been my happiest time.' It was there he met his wife, a librarian working in London. 'I thought the

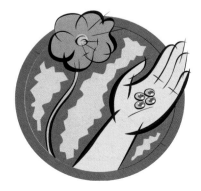

English had their priorities right. They studied medicine for the right reasons. Within the national health service, there is a much more ethical and moral approach to medicine.'

His departure was not, he says, to do with the shocking discoveries he made when he decided to look into the history of the Vienna medical school for a special occasion. He found the official records stopped in 1938. He was told he had better not delve further, but in a paper that he describes as among the most important he has ever published, in the *Annals of Internal Medicine* of May 1995, Ernst exposed the terrible truth of what took place during the Nazi years in the name of medicine in Vienna.

Jewish doctors who dominated the profession there were sacked – 153 of the 197 faculty members – and the dean was replaced by the Nazi professor Eduard Pernkopf. Appalling atrocities took place. Many children were killed at the paediatric hospital. Pernkopf worked on an anatomical atlas, which is still in use, drawn from the bodies of those children, and his institute of anatomy used the corpses of the executed for teaching. Viennese professors led experiments on prisoners at Dachau. After the war the Jewish doctors who had been sacked but survived were not invited back, and the Nazi physicians stayed on, mostly escaping retribution.

In a letter in a later edition of the journal, Ernst wrote: 'It is important to realise that, by and large, the German and Austrian medical professions were not victimised by the Nazis but actively guided the developments leading to the monstrous disasters and unspeakable violations of ethical behaviour.' His family was not Jewish and his father had a clean record in the war, but Ernst finds it hard to deal with the legacy of medicine under the Nazis. He has no wish to return to Germany and he has taken British nationality, 'because it became clear to me that this is where I will spend my days. It is just an honest way of approaching it.'

There have been several tempting offers from the US, where he has quite a following. 'For a long time, I loved going over to America because they would fall over with admiration there. I felt so flattered.'

He admits to 'several sleepless nights' but finally turned them down. After all, at least a third of the reason for taking the job was to come to England, he says.

Looking through a summary of the mountain of papers his unit has published in 10 years, a lesser mortal might feel discouraged. Most of the findings on the efficacy of therapies and treatments are either negative or inconclusive because too little research has been done for anyone to be sure. But not Ernst.

'They are not always negative results. In meta analyses [pooling the results of all available good quality studies], we generate quite a lot of positive results,' he says.

Herbs such as St John's wort, which has proved effective in treating depression, have shown much promise. Kava kava also proved effective in relieving anxiety. But then evidence surfaced linking it to liver damage.

'I fought very hard not to have it banned,' says Ernst, who has been on the Medicines Commission in the UK since his Vienna days. 'I thought that the argument of the authorities neglected the efficacy side of it totally. I felt that the risk was being addressed in isolation. There was a risk and it needed addressing. To forget about it would have been totally wrong, but an outright ban on it was harsh.

'I have often said that if you banned kava today, you should have banned Valium ten years ago.' (Kava kava has been voluntarily withdrawn from sale in the UK, pending a formal legal ban.)

Among his successes, he numbers the study of the safety of acupuncture, which he carried out against the mass opposition of acupuncturists, who clearly thought he was out to get them. They needed 30,000 patients, he calculated, to make it definitive. He managed to get the doctors practising acupuncture on board, and the rest did their own study on a similar model. They found a very small percentage of very mild adverse events.

'All of a sudden we became the heroes of the acupuncture world,' he says. 'The lesson is that studying safety is not to the detriment necessarily of complementary medicine.

'We are likely to show that it is safer than whatever else is used for that condition, but safety is too important an issue to leave to assumption or public opinion.'

'People mistakenly think I must be a promoter of complementary medicine – that I should have an allegiance to the camp. I don't. My allegiance is firstly to the patient'

His biggest frustration is over the lack of funding for the research he wants to do. It matters. A quarter of the population and close to 100% of cancer patients use complementary medicine, and yet 0.5% of charitable funds and 0.8% of NHS grants go to CAM studies. 'That to me is pretty outrageous.'

They have submitted more than 200 grant applications and roughly one in 20 is funded. 'I'm a pretty tough guy and highly motivated, but when the young researchers have been turned down three or four times I find it hard to motivate anybody.'

He is scathing about the grant review panels who reject applications because his researchers cannot use standardised doses of their therapies. 'They are demonstrating that they are reviewing applications they should not be reviewing in the first place,' he says.

Maurice Laing's 10-year funding runs out in October. Laing has agreed to pay for three more years. The unit is a world leader and has recently become part of the Peninsula medical school in Exeter – enormous achievements, but Ernst still has a precarious future, and, at 55, no Viennese pension to look forward to. Does he regret taking the job on?

'Not for one minute,' he says. 'There were milliseconds at the very beginning when I thought, what have I done, particularly coming from a pompous, big institution. But a lot of money that they were throwing at me in Vienna doesn't necessarily make for good doctoring or good science.'

© Guardian Newspapers Limited 2003

Reasons for using CAM

A BBC Radio 5 Live survey, reported by Ernst & White, asked 245 CAM users what their reason were for using CAM.

Reasons	No.	%
1. Helps relieve injury/condition	60	24.5
2. Just like it	51	20.8
3. Find it relaxing	46	18.8
4. For good health/wellbeing	34	13.9
5. Preventative	30	12.2
6. Don't believe in conventional medicine	27	11.0
7. Doctor's referral	27	11.0
8. Find out about other ways of life	26	10.6
9. Way of life/lifestyle	20	8.2
10. Can't get NHS treatment	17	6.9
11. Exercise	5	2.0
12. To meet other people/make friends	2	0.8
13. Other	15	6.1
14. Don't know/not sure	9	3.7

These reponses are problematic in that this survey does not distinguish between over-the-counter purchases, practitioner interventions or classes, such as yoga or t'ai chi.

Source: Ernst & White 2000, The Prince of Wales's Foundation for Integrated Health

Hands-on healing, or a con?

What do scientists think about 'alternative' therapies?

By Orla Kennedy

Is complementary medicine hocus-pocus or does it warrant large-scale scientific investigation? Should science range beyond conventional medicine and conduct research on alternative medicine and the supposed growing links between mind and body? This was hotly debated at the British Association for the Advancement of Science in Salford 10 September 2003.

One Briton in five uses complementary medicine, and according to the most recent Mintel survey, one in 10 uses herbalism or homeopathy. Around £130 million is spent on oils, potions and pills every year in Britain, and the complementary and alternative medicine industry is estimated to be worth £1.6 billion.

With the help of Professor Edzard Ernst, Laing chair of complementary medicine at the Peninsula Medical School, Universities of Exeter and Plymouth, The *Daily Telegraph* asked scientists their views on complementary and alternative medicine. Seventy-five scientists, in fields ranging from molecular biology to neuroscience, replied.

Surprisingly, our sample of scientists was twice as likely as the public to use some form of complementary medicine, at around four in 10 compared with two in 10 of the general population. Three-quarters of scientific users believed they were effective. Acupuncture, chiropractic and osteopathy were the most commonly used complementary treatments among scientists and more than 55 per cent believed these were more effective than a placebo and should be available to all on the NHS.

Scientists appear to place more trust in the more established areas of complementary and alternative medicine, such as acupuncture, chiropractic and osteopathy, for which there are professional bodies and recognised training, than therapies such as aromatherapy and spiritual healing.

'Osteopathy is now a registered profession requiring a certified four-year degree before you can advertise as an osteopath and practise,' said one neuroscientist who used the therapy.

> *Around £130 million is spent on oils, potions and pills every year in Britain, and the complementary and alternative medicine industry is estimated to be worth £1.6 billion*

Nearly two thirds of the scientists who replied to our survey believed that aromatherapy and homeopathy were no better than placebos, with almost a half thinking the same of herbalism and spiritual healing.

Some of the comments we received were scathing, even though one in 10 of our respondents had used homeopathy. 'Aromatherapy and homeopathy are scientifically non-sensical,' said one molecular biologist from the University of Bristol.

Dr Romke Bron, a molecular biologist at the Medical Research Council Centre for Developmental Neurobiology at King's College London, added: 'Homeopathy is a big scam and I am convinced that if someone would sneak into a homeopathic pharmacy and swap labels, nobody would notice anything.'

In homeopathy, 'like cures like'. That is why hallucinogenic toadstools that make you twitch supposedly treat twitching. And 'the most effective dose is the minimum dose'. Whole live wolf spiders and deadly nightshade are among the ingredients used to make a 'mother tincture', which is mixed with water in a series of 1:100 dilutions so that at the '12th potency', the possibility that one molecule remains is remote.

Two centuries after homeopathy was introduced, it still lacks a watertight demonstration that it works. Scientists are happy that the resulting solutions and sugar pills have no side effects, but are baffled by how they can do anything. Yet, of

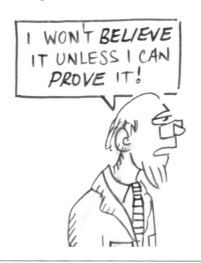

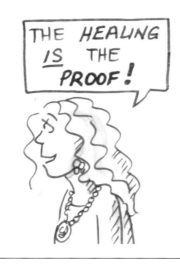

the small number of scientists surveyed who had taken homeopathic medicines, most thought they had worked.

Both complementary and conventional medicine should be used in routine health care, according to followers of the 'integrated health approach', who want to treat an individual 'as a whole'.

The Prince of Wales, one of the leading lights in this area, has set up his own Foundation for Integrated Health. He said recently that 'in the complex health-care world of the 21st century, no single therapeutic practice could possibly have a monopoly on effective diagnosis and treatment for all conditions. Scientific, psychological, nutritional, environmental and spiritual insights must surely be fully employed to restore and maintain health.'

But the scientists who responded to our survey expressed serious concerns about this approach, with more than half believing that integrated medicine was an attempt to bypass rigorous scientific testing. Scientists thought that although this strategy was politically correct, it was scientifically flawed.

Dr Bron said: 'There is an awful lot of bad science going on in alternative medicine and the general public has a hard time to distinguish between scientific myth and fact.

'It is absolutely paramount to maintain rigorous quality control in health care. Although the majority of alternative health workers mean well, there are just too many frauds out there preying on vulnerable people.'

The House of Lords select committee on science and technology's report on complementary and alternative medicine in 2000 recommended better regulation and research into this area so that both the public and the medical establishment have confidence in its effectiveness and safety. The Government's five-year programme providing £7.5 million for research in complementary medicine is about to begin.

One molecular biologist from the University of Warwick admitted that 'by doing this poll I have realised how shamefully little I understand about alternative therapy. Not

Complementary and alternative treatments

Acupuncture: fine needles are inserted at special points along 'meridians' or 'energy' centres.

Aromatherapy uses aromatic, volatile oils of plants, usually applied through gentle massage.

Chiropractic involves manual treatment of the spine and extremities using sometimes high velocity thrusts.

Herbalism uses herbs that contain a range of pharmacologically active ingredients.

Homeopathy (see main article). Massage is kneading, stroking and pummelling of muscles and connective tissue to achieve relaxation and increased circulation and wellbeing.

Osteopathy is similar to chiropractic but usually gentler.

Spiritual healing is the channelling of energies by the healer to re-energise the patient.

Yoga uses postural, stretching and breathing exercises, meditation and other techniques.

enough scientific research has been performed. There is enough anecdotal evidence to suggest that at least some of the therapies are effective for some people, suggesting this is an area ripe for research.'

When asked if complementary and alternative medicine should get more research funding, scientists believed the top three (acupuncture, chiropractic and osteopathy) should get money, as should herbalism. It seems that therapies based on physical manipulation or a known action – like the active ingredients

---

Both complementary and conventional medicine should be used in routine health care, according to followers of the 'integrated health approach'

---

in a herb on a receptor in the body – are the ones that the scientific community has faith in.

Less than a quarter thought that therapies such as aromatherapy, homeopathy and spiritual healing should get any funding. In the current cash-strapped climate of the NHS, it was felt that funding was more urgently needed for day-to-day services and research into 'real' medical problems.

Scientists believed that the 'feelgood' counselling effect of complementary medicine and the time taken to listen to patients' problems was what worked, rather than any medicinal effect. In contrast, the average GP visit lasts only eight minutes, says the British Medical Association.

Dr Stephen Nurrish, a molecular biologist at University College London, said: 'As GPs become business managers, the time they spend with patients becomes less and less. Much of the benefit people get from complementary medicine is the time to talk to someone and be listened to sympathetically, something that is now lacking from "Western" medicine.'

But an anonymous neuroscientist at King's College London had a more withering view of this benefit: 'On the validity of complementary and alternative medicines, no one would dispute that "feeling good" is good for your health, but why discriminate between museum-trip therapy, patting-a-dog therapy and aromatherapy? Is it because only the latter has a cadre of professional "practitioners"?'

There are other hardline scientists who argue that there should be no such thing as complementary and alternative medicine. As Professor David Moore, director of the Medical Research Council's Institute for Hearing Research, said: 'Either a treatment works or it doesn't. The only way to determine if it works is to test it against appropriate controls (that is, scientifically).'

If you want to find out more about the British Association's annual festival, see its web site at www.the-ba.net

Alternative therapies win NHS backing

Government watchdog breaks new ground by giving cautious endorsement of some complementary medicines in treating multiple sclerosis

The role of complementary therapies such as fish oils, reflexology and t'ai chi in treating disease are recognised for the first time in official NHS guidance published 25 November 2003.

The cautious and still only partial endorsement of the possible benefits from such treatments in easing the symptoms of multiple sclerosis comes from the government's clinical watchdog for England and Wales, the National Institute for Clinical Excellence (Nice).

Complementary treatments are widely used by patients with the progressive, incurable disease. Even this small step by Nice is a significant recognition of the avenues pursued by patients desperate to find relief from pain, fatigue and other symptoms.

It is understood that another clinical guideline expected soon – for treating depression – will also acknowledge a place for complementary therapy.

The MS guidelines, aimed at health professionals, still leave much of the onus and risk from complementary medicine – both medical and financial – on individual patients.

By James Meikle, Health Correspondent

However, it will mean that doctors raise the issue of alternative treatments with patients early on.

It says patients should be informed that there is 'some evidence to suggest' that some might have benefits, even if there is not enough evidence to make firm recommendations.

As well as fish oils, massage and t'ai chi, the treatments include magnetic field therapy, where the patient lies on a pad fixed behind the spine and linked by cable to a computer-controlled bedside unit.

> **There is no endorsement for other non-orthodox treatments, such as acupuncture, yoga, herbal remedies or aromatherapy**

Neural therapy, involving local anaesthetics to clear up 'electrical interference', is another option that might work. So is massage and multi-modal therapy, an educational and psychological approach.

But there is no endorsement for other non-orthodox treatments, such as acupuncture, yoga, herbal remedies or aromatherapy. And in all cases, patients should be encouraged to tell doctors if they decide to pursue complementary treatments.

The Multiple Sclerosis Society has two concerns about complementary medicine: that it is used safely and that patients are not overcharged. Such treatment is not usually available on the NHS, and patients often have to bear the costs themselves. The society's leaflet on the issue advises caution.

'Trying everything can be very expensive and demoralising,' it says. 'If a therapy does not work for you, or you start to feel worse, you may end up feeling that it's your own fault.'

Much of the problem is that MS fluctuates and is unpredictable. The Nice guidelines do not mention cannabis-based medicines. Recently published results from a large trial suggested that these might benefit patients, despite an absence of objective evidence of improvement. Nice is to fast-track a review of these if such drugs are granted a licence by

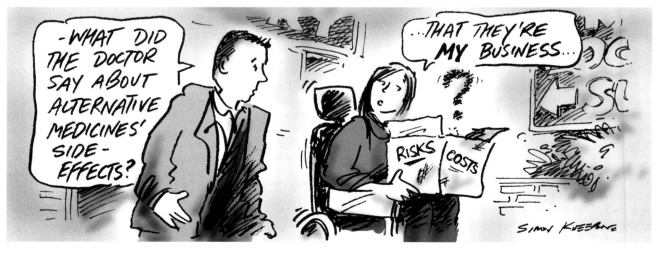

another government body which controls use of medicines.

The more mainstream advice in the guidelines calls for rapid diagnosis, preferably well within three months after first referral to a consultant, more specialised services and primary care by GPs to recognise particular problems faced by MS patients, including depression and sexual dysfunction. The diagnosis target will require a huge increase in neurologists to deliver results.

Patient groups welcomed the guidelines, arguing that thousands of people among the estimated 63,000 with MS in England and Wales suffered from a healthcare lottery, although examples of good practice are found in a number of places, including London, Merseyside and Newcastle.

Which treatments are sanctioned?

In
T'ai chi
Ancient Chinese form of body movement focusing on development of internal energy to promote physical and mental wellbeing. Long advocated for tackling heart, breathing and digestive problems as well as relieving stress

Magnetic field therapy
Treatment advertised by US companies as effective against all sorts of pain, including arthritis, osteoporosis and sports injuries. Also promoted as treatment for cats, dogs and horses

Massage
Stimulates blood flow round the body and helps relaxation. Can cause muscles to go into spasm, so not all patients will benefit

Reflexology
Foot massage to stimulate healing in other parts of the body

Out
Magnetic bracelets
Sometimes used to prevent tremors by MS patients, but no conclusive research base, and when bought over the counter are not tailored to meet specific needs, according to MS Society

Meditation
Focus on the moment and clear the mind to counteract negative thinking. No endorsement from new guidance

Breathing oxygen in pressurised chamber
Available at some MS therapy centres, but can be expensive as well as potentially dangerous. It has some real fans, but some other patients report a worsening of symptoms

Jury still out
Cannabis-based drugs
Helps feelgood factor and eases symptoms, according to patients in recent trials, despite lack of hard objective evidence that they ease muscle stiffness.

However, signs are that the government will endorse their use if medicines watchdogs are happy about safety and effectiveness.

© Guardian Newspapers Limited 2003

Building confidence in CAM

Complementary and alternative medicine will become more widely accepted and thus available to those in need when there is solid evidence to answer three questions

Is it safe?
With virtually all therapies, direct and indirect risks exist. Compared to mainstream medicine, CAM is probably associated with far fewer risks. However, we need to find out how often side effects or complications happen.

Examples:
1. After monitoring 30,000 acupuncture treatments, our researchers have demonstrated conclusively that this form of treatment is safe.
2. An analysis of all randomised clinical trials and other studies has shown that the medicinal herb Kava is effective in reducing anxiety.

Is it effective?
To CAM providers, effectiveness is obvious. Yet its success can be due to several factors – specific therapeutic effect, time spent with the patient, placebo effect, and natural history of the disease, etc. Our researchers aim to differentiate between these elements.

Examples:
1. An analysis of clinical trials has demonstrated that horse chestnut seed extracts are an effective treatment to alleviate the symptoms of varicose veins.
2. Ginkgo biloba is more effective than placebo, and as effective as conventional medication, in prolonging the walking distance of patients with peripheral arterial disease.

Is it value for money?
Most CAM providers take it for granted that complementary and alternative medicine saves cost. There is, however, the possibility that CAM is an 'add-on' expense within the healthcare system. At a time when rationing of costs has become a major issue, we need to find out the truth. Only proper cost-evaluation methodology will answer this question.

■ The above information is from Complementary Medicine's web site which can be found at www.pms.ac.uk/compmed/

© Complementary Medicine at the Universities of Exeter & Plymouth

Complementary and alternative therapies

Information from Cancer Research UK

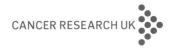

The phrases 'complementary therapy' and 'alternative therapy' are often used as if they meant the same thing. But there is an important difference: complementary therapies are used alongside conventional medical treatments. Some of them have been scientifically tested and can be useful to help patients relax and cope with stress, pain and side effects of standard cancer treatment.

Alternative therapies are more often used instead of conventional medical treatment. Some alternative therapists claim to be able to cure cancer even if conventional medical treatments have not been able to cure it. These alternative cures have not usually been tested scientifically in clinical trials. We do not know whether they will help slow the growth of cancer. Many are harmless, but others may cause strong side effects, or involve unnecessarily invasive procedures. In any case, aborting or withholding standard, scientifically tested cancer treatments can deprive patients of the best possible chance of successful treatment or relief of symptoms.

Of those complementary treatments that can be beneficial, not all are suitable for all patients all of the time. Patients should always talk to their doctor before deciding whether to have complementary treatment. The doctor can explain to patients why for their specific cancer some forms may be better than others.

On this subject, Dr Richard Sullivan, Head of Clinical Programmes for Cancer Research UK, said (abridged):

'Treatments for cancer have a long history of evidence behind them. Doctors carry out clinical trials comparing the standard treatments with the new ones to see which one is really better. It's this approach since the 1950s that means in the UK alone over 100,000 people a year are treated successful for cancer. 7 out 10 ten children now survive cancer with modern chemotherapy; 50 years ago nearly 90% died. Death rates from breast cancer have fallen by 22% in the last ten years thanks to the combination of screening, better surgery, new chemotherapy and the endocrine treatment tamoxifen. 95% of men are cured of their testicular cancer with chemotherapy. All of these facts come out of research and evidence-based medicine as a result of proper clinical trials to ensure that there really is a good basis for treatment. This is the type of information that cancer doctors have at their disposal when they give cancer patients the various treatment options.

Some patients choose complementary or alternative therapies in addition to modern medical treatment

---

'Everyone though has an absolute right to decide how he or she wants to be treated for cancer. Cancer specialists draw on years of training and decades of solid evidence to offer patients the right treatment. There is always a choice to be treated or not. Sometimes a choice between different treatments. Some patients choose complementary or alternative therapies in addition to modern medical treatment. How-ever, the plain fact remains that only modern cancer treatments have ever been proven to cure or delay cancer. That's not to say that complementary therapies don't have a role in alleviating some of the symptoms of cancer or its treatment, it's just that I wouldn't bet my life on it if I had cancer.'

Evidence on specific regimes

1. 'Breuss Cancer Cure'
There is no evidence that this dietary regime has any positive effect on cancer. Its aim to starve the cancer of protein could potentially lead to malnutrition, which may impede the body's resistance to cancer.

2. Laetrile
Laetrile has shown very little anti-cancer activity in laboratory experiments, and no effects in human trials. Use of laetrile can, however, lead to severe and potentially lethal cyanide poisoning.

3. Mind/Body techniques
These can help patients in alleviating symptoms and promoting psychological well-being alongside standard cancer treatments.

4. Homeopathy
There is some evidence that homeopathy can help relieve symptoms of cancer therapy. Homoeopathy is being used in certain NHS hospitals alongside standard treatment.

5. Mistletoe
Despite promising effects in some laboratory studies, there is to date no evidence that mistletoe extract can slow or cure cancer in humans.

6. Gerson therapy
While trying to maintain a balanced

diet can help cancer patients, to date there is no evidence that this regime, which was initially developed against headaches, has any positive effect on cancer. A stringent dietary regime and multiple daily enemas are arduous and expensive.

7. Traditional Chinese medicine
This is a complex topic, and there is some evidence from studies that certain herbs or herbal extracts can help relieve side effects of cancer treatments. Several important cancer drugs in current use were derived from plants, and there is considerable interest in the identification and purification of further phyto-medicines active against cancer. However, some plants and plant products can be very toxic, especially when taken in unusually large quantities. Patients should seek advice before using uncommon herbs or herbal extracts.

8. Acupuncture
As in Mind/Body.

9. Shiitake mushrooms
These have shown promising effects in stimulating the immune system to fight disease and reducing side effects from cancer treatment. They cannot, however, replace standard cancer treatments. What also needs to be established is whether studies done in the Far East were of similarly rigorous standards as those practised in the West.

10. Ayurveda
Meditation and breathing exercises may have similar beneficial effects to acupuncture and mind/body therapies on patient's well-being. Some herbs and herbal extracts used in Ayurveda may have useful anti-cancer properties. However, studies have not progressed far enough to tell.

11. Cancer salves (Escharotics)
There is no evidence that such preparations can slow or cure cancer. Ingredients such as zinc oxide are corrosive and can cause skin damage, making these preparations unsuitable for anyone.

12. Essiac tea
The is no evidence of an anti-cancer

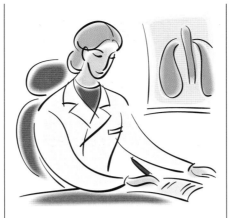

effect of this tea. Patients should – as with all unusual foods and food supplements – talk to their doctor about whether it might be useful to improve well-being.

13. Pau D'Arco tea
While some laboratory studies suggest effects against soft tissue tumours, the medical literature reports severe side effects of this tea. It should therefore not be used unless further studies can confirm its safety.

14. Oxygen therapy
Professor Peter Wardman, Head of the Cancer Research UK Free Radicals Research Group, said: 'Ozone is a highly reactive gas with the potential to damage many biological molecules. At very low levels in some model systems it can inactivate harmful species or stimulate the immune system, along with the destruction of natural anti-oxidants that would be one of the first effects of ozone exposure.

'However, the possibility of benefit to humans from exposure to ozone seems to me to be far outweighed by the possibility of detriment. Most of the claims seem unsubstantiated by randomised clinical trials. I would describe a suggestion that ozone exposure might be considered as a preventative treatment for cancer as "absurd". Individuals should not consider such treatment in the context of cancer.

'The biological effects of ozone are quite unrelated to the implications of varying oxygen levels in tumours, a topic which Cancer Research UK scientists are actively researching.'

15. Gonzalez protocol
The study mentioned does not seem to have progressed far enough to evaluate the benefits and effects of this dietary regimen.

16. Shark cartilage
Trials so far have provided inconclusive results (and sharks do get cancer). The current studies will add to our knowledge, which may enable us to tell whether components of shark cartilage could be useful to shut down tumour blood vessels.

17. Kombucha
There is no evidence to suggest an anti-cancer effect. However, some studies have reported toxic side effects, making it an unsuitable supplement alongside cancer treatment.

18. Aromatherapy
Aromatherapy can assist by improving patients' well-being during and after cancer treatment.

19. Orthomolecular oncology
There is no evidence that the very high doses of supplements proposed have beneficial effects. At these levels, overdoses of fat-soluble vitamins and other supplements are possible. There is also evidence for pro-cancer effects of some supplements. High intake of vitamin A in smokers increases lung cancer risk.

20. PC-SPES
PC-SPES has been pulled from the market in the US over fears of warfarin content, which could lead to excessive bleeding in some people. Trials are under way, and so far there have been some promising effects reported as well as potentially severe side effects.

Further studies are needed to establish the safety of PC-SPES and assess any potential benefits.

■ The above information is from Cancer Research UK, for further information visit their web site at www.cancerresearch.org.uk Alternatively, see their address details on page 41.
© Cancer Research UK

Why bogus therapies seem to work

There is a website worth visiting if you are concerned about the benefits or otherwise of alternative therapies (www.quackwatch.com), but note that Bandolier does not endorse the contents of the site or its conclusions. One page is devoted to why 'bogus' therapies seem to work. The points are well made and some apply just as much to conventional as alternative therapies. Most of the points are where non-scientific belief can be nullified by proper scientific method.

That is the main reason why high quality studies of alternative therapies are negative, while lower quality studies are positive. If bias exists in the usual clinical situation, it is even more relevant for alternative therapies where belief in the value of the therapy is very strong.

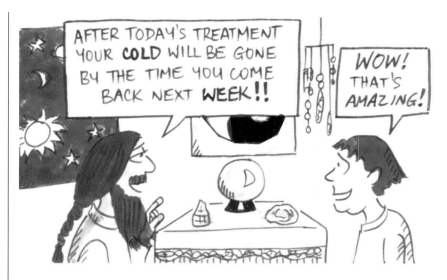

Many diseases are self-limiting

The old saying is that a cold will go away in a week or in seven days if you treat it. Determining whether an intervention has made a difference is therefore difficult. Unless rigorous study methods are applied, an apparent benefit cannot be ascribed to the intervention or the natural course of the disease.

Many diseases are cyclical

Allergies, multiple sclerosis, arthritis and gastrointestinal problems like irritable bowel syndrome all have their ups and downs. Sufferers may seek therapy on a down, so that when an up comes that has to be due to the therapy, doesn't it? Again, only rigorous study design combats this.

Placebo effect

Both the above contribute to what is called a placebo effect. It can be seen as the natural course of things. For instance, some people need no pain relief after surgery,[1] making a preemptive intervention which claims to reduce pain after surgery a sure win. There will always be some people publicly to declaim its value. Natural 'placebo' rates depend on what the problem is and what the benefit is. There will always be some people who benefit without an intervention.

Bets are 'hedged'

'My auntie was under the doctor for six months, but it was only when she started on homeopathy that she got better.' The fact that the poor infantry slaved away for six months is forgotten in the glamour of magic.

Original diagnosis may be wrong

Bandolier has highlighted the difficulty of diagnosis. If the diagnosis is wrong, then miraculous cures are less miraculous.

Alternative healers often have much more time to spend with their patient than a harassed GP loaded down with kilograms of guidelines and tight budgets

---

Mood improvement or cure

Alternative healers often have much more time to spend with their patient than a harassed GP loaded down with kilograms of guidelines and tight prescribing budgets. Is it any wonder that alternative healers can make patients feel better? That mood change is sometimes seen as the cure.

Psychological investment in alternatives

Alternative healing can be as simple as some herbal remedy bought from a shop. Sometimes it can involve huge amounts of time, massive involvement of the family, and an intense psychological investment in believing that something (anything) will work. It is not surprising, then, that many people find some redeeming value in the treatment.

Reference
1   HJ McQuay, RES Bullingham, RA Moore, PJD Evans, JW Lloyd. Some patients don't need analgesics after surgery. *Journal of the Royal Society of Medicine* 1982 75, 705-708.

■ The above information is from Bandolier's web site which can be found at www.jr2.ox.ac.uk/bandolier/index.html

An iguana a day keeps the doctor away?

Even the most diehard supporters of trendy health supplements might find it hard to swallow a lizard!

In a shocking survey of 2,000 carried out by The Nutri Centre @ Tesco:

- A staggering 65% of people who took part admitted they 'weren't entirely sure' of the ingredients of the complementary health supplements they were buying.
- 68% of the general public revealed that they thought that Iguana was a digestive aid or a herbal cough remedy rather than a lizard.
- 75% have found the names of the supplements confusing.
- 6 out of 9 products were wrongly identified against a multiple choice of supposed treatment areas.
- 68% who don't currently take complementary health products would do so if they had a clearer idea of which ones to use.

This frightening level of confusion over alternative health products highlights the need for retailers to take a more responsible stance in helping educate their customers on complementary health choices.

The Nutri Centre @ Tesco is committed to helping everyone get the best from complementary health rather than be confused by the terminology.

Karen Simister, Category Manager for Healthcare at Tesco, commented, 'It really doesn't surprise me that 68% thought that an Iguana was a herbal remedy rather than a large lizard!

'The complementary health market is exploding at the moment as more and more people become aware of the reported benefits of vitamins, minerals and other alternative supplements. What can often happen, however, is that consumers find themselves overwhelmed when they are faced with the shelves of strangely named products.

'At The Nutri Centre @ Tesco we are committed to helping our customers choose the right products through clear labelling and naming of our products. We have recently launched a new range that is easy to select from, as each product is clearly named by its benefit e.g. "Energy Support", "Immune Support", "Hair, Skin and Nail Support" etc.

68% of the general public revealed that they thought that Iguana was a digestive aid or a herbal cough remedy rather than a lizard

---

'The supplements are careful blends of the recommended vitamins, minerals and herbal supplements to give the best possible complementary solutions for key health issues. We do not believe in confusing our customers, we want to help them get the most from complementary medicine and our survey showed that 89% of the public wanted clearer labelling of alternative health products.'

Other results from the survey include:

- 35% of the general public revealed that they take complementary supplements without really understanding what they are supposed to do for them.
- 52% would buy complementary health products on the back of a newspaper or magazine recommendation.
- 18% would buy products because they believed that celebrities took them.

The Nutri Centre @ Tesco Complementary Health range comprises 13 products including Milk Thistle, Bone Support, Immune Support and Energy Support. The range is available from The Nutri Centre @ Tesco fixtures in more than 200 of the top Tesco stores. To find out where your nearest is call 0800 505 555 or for further information visit www.tesco.com

© *Tesco*
December, 2003

Mean expenditure

A BBC Radio 5 Live survey, reported by Ernst & White (2000), identified that 60% of CAM expenditure per month was £10 or less and that the mean expenditure for all respondents was £13.62. This translates to an estimated average annual expenditure of £163.44.

	Mean expenditure per month
All	£13.62
Sex	
Male	£13.11
Female	£13.96
Age group	
18-24	£18.61
25-34	£15.57
35-64	£12.56
65+	£13.29

Source: Ernst & White 2000, The Prince of Wales's Foundation for Integrated Health

Setting the agenda for the future

Information from the Prince of Wales's Foundation for Integrated Health

What is integrated health?

Integrated medicine or healthcare is not another term for complementary medicine, nor does it represent an alternative to conventional care. An integrated approach is much wider. It focuses on health and healing, rather than just disease and treatment and seeks to bring together body, mind and spirit so that healthcare encompasses the whole person. Integrated healthcare sees each human being as an individual and starts by recognising that each one of us has many dimensions and lives in a unique social and environmental context. It acknowledges the high level of responsibility individuals have for their own health.

The concept of integrated health 'involves patients and doctors working to maintain health by paying attention to lifestyle factors such as diet, exercise, quality of rest and sleep, and the nature of relationships,' wrote Dr Andrew Weil, director of the integrative medicine programme at Arizona University and Professor Dame Lesley Rees, the Foundation's new chair, in the *British Medical Journal* in January 2001.[1]

In such a partnership, conventional and complementary practitioners would work together. For example, a physician might prescribe medication for migraine, but look for underlying factors such as stress or diet that could cause or perpetuate the condition. An integrated therapeutic package agreed with the patient and with complementary practitioners could include acupuncture to reduce the frequency of attacks and induce relaxation, nutritional advice, a herbal remedy as a preventive measure and yoga, relaxation and other stress-management techniques to encourage natural healing processes.

Twenty-first-century healthcare is complex and no single professional therapeutic practice can possibly have the monopoly of effective diagnosis and treatment for all conditions. Increasing awareness by healthcare professionals who work together is called for, so that scientific, psychological, nutritional, environmental and spiritual insights may be employed together to fully restore and maintain health.

Such a challenge needs facilitation, and dedicated fundraising, encouragement and inspiration. The Foundation is well placed for such a task.

Increasing use of complementary medicine

Complementary medicine has enjoyed a considerable rise in popularity over the last twenty years, which clearly suggests that people are interested in taking responsibility for their own health and well-being.

> The concept of integrated health 'involves patients and doctors working to maintain health'

A 1998 survey conducted by the University of Sheffield's Medical Care Research Unit found that 10.6% of the adult population had visited at least one practitioner providing acupuncture, chiropractic, homeopathy, medical herbalism, hypnotherapy or osteopathy in the previous year. If aromatherapy and reflexology were included, the figure increased to 13.6%.[2]

The survey showed that 79% of these visits were paid for directly by the patient, an expenditure of £580 million. That people are prepared to pay themselves is an indication of the value they place on their health. By comparison, the NHS paid an estimated £50-55 million in the same period for the provision of complementary medicine in the NHS, mainly for orthopaedic or cancer patients.

In a BBC Radio 5 Live survey in 1999, about 25% of respondents said they had used or experienced complementary therapies at some time. Perhaps even more significantly, 74% said they would choose complementary therapies if they were available in the NHS.[3]

Self-care

Anecdotal evidence suggests that individuals are already integrating

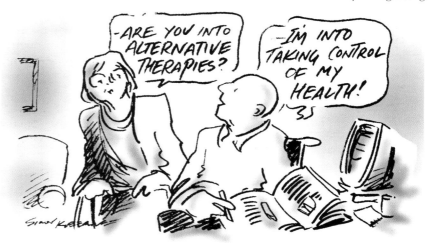

conventional and complementary medicine for themselves. At the first sign of a cold, for example, many people will routinely self-dose with echinacea, a herb claimed to have immunity-boosting properties. They may take vitamin C with or without zinc, nutrients said to enhance production of infection-fighting white cells. If these measures fail, then conventional over-the-counter preparations of aspirin, paracetamol and ibuprofen are the next resort, along with various decongestants, cough suppressants and even old-fashioned steam inhalations.

Figures for the sales of nutritional supplements and herbal remedies are also buoyant. The BBC survey showed that those using complementary medicine spent on average £14 a month in paying practitioners and buying products, about £1.6 billion a year. Industry sources estimated that the market for herbal and homeopathic medicines and aromatherapy essential oils was worth £109 million in 2000 and predicted a rise to £126 million in 2002.

Consumer choice

Why are people turning to complementary medicine? A number of reasons have been proposed. There is an increasing degree of disenchantment with conventional medicine and the way in which it is delivered. Improved living standards and mass inoculation programmes in the 20th century, combined with life-saving medical and scientific breakthroughs such as antibiotics and other miracle drugs, MRI scans, keyhole surgery and gene therapy, have raised expectations of health and healthcare.

However, there are increasing concerns about potential side effects to drugs and the growing resistance to antibiotics. Confidence in conventional medicine has also been eroded by the seemingly frustrating progress in finding a cure for cancer and AIDS. In addition, there are long waiting times for specialist appointments and a perception that doctors have little to offer for a wide range of disabling chronic conditions. All this has lead people to look at other healthcare options.

At least 40% of general practices in the UK provide some form of complementary services

Under the NHS Britons may be more constrained in their choice of GP and consultant than patients with private insurance in the United States or Australia, but the notion of shopping around for healthcare has taken hold. Those who can afford it have the choice of a wide range of over-the-counter medicines, nutritional supplements and herbal remedies and of complementary practitioners. As a result, many have come to regard themselves as active partners in their healthcare and expect a personal approach and a positive relationship with their healthcare practitioner.[4]

Medical attitudes

The attitude of the medical profession to complementary therapies has shifted almost seismically since 1980, when the British Medical Association compared chiropractic to the 'examination of a bird's entrails' and described acupuncturists' beliefs as irrational.[5,6] Only two decades later the BMA published a report on acupuncture, which stated that 79% of GPs would like to see acupuncture available on the NHS,[7] and in 2001 the British Medical Journal devoted a substantial section of an entire issue to integrated medicine.[8]

At least 40% of general practices in the UK provide some form of complementary services,[9] while unofficially many more refer patients who can pay to private complementary practitioners. But, as over 90% of complementary healthcare is purchased privately, the benefits of this integrated approach may only be available to those who can pay.

The need for guidance

In response to the increased use by the public of complementary medicine and practitioners, the House of Lords Select Committee on Science and Technology made a 15-month study of complementary and alternative medicine, publishing its report in November 2000.[10]

Its conclusions were trenchant. Research into whether the therapies worked needed to be encouraged. Training courses varied unacceptably in content, depth and duration. Regulation of the many different specialities was fragmented and inadequate. 'There is a clear need for more effective guidance for the public as to what does or does not work and what is or is not safe in CAM,' said the report.

If integrated healthcare is to achieve what many health practitioners are coming to see as its considerable therapeutic potential, then sympathetic, even-handed and influential leadership is essential. This is a natural role for the Foundation, with its programme of encouraging evidence-based research, steering practitioners towards improved regulation and training standards, supporting interdisciplinary collaboration and disseminating information.

Setting the scene
The first five years

In 1997 the Foundation published the discussion document Integrated Healthcare: A Way Forward for the Next Five Years? This examined practical ways in which conventional and complementary health practitioners could develop a working partnership. It set out the basis of an integrated healthcare system that:

- encouraged patients to be actively involved in their own health care and treatment
- combined the best of conventional and complementary medicine

His Royal Highness The Prince of Wales, together with Mr Frank Dobson, then Secretary of State for Health, launched this programme at a groundbreaking conference in May 1998. Many senior figures in conventional and complementary medicine met for the first time and established mutual areas of interest.

Key objectives identified as vital in achieving integrated healthcare were education, information, regulation, research and development and delivery. Over the last five years, the Foundation has worked at national and local levels to develop an extensive programme of work in these areas. In the same period, the NHS has undergone major changes in funding and organisation. In November 2000 the House of Lords Select Committee on Science and Technology published its report on complementary and alternative medicine. This report closely mirrored the Foundation's objectives, set out in its 1997 discussion document.

The select committee report called for more evidence-based research, tighter regulation of therapies and practitioners, and more information to enable the public to make an informed choice of health-care. Four months later, in March 2001, the government accepted the report's recommendations.[11]

References

1 Rees, L, Weil, A. Integrated medicine. *BMJ* 2001; 322: 119-120.
2 Thomas KJ, Nicholl JP, Coleman P. Use and expenditure on complementary medicine in England: a population based survey. *Complementary Therapies in Medicine* 2001, 9: 2-11.
3 Ernst E, White A. The BBC survey of complementary medicine use in the UK. *Complementary Therapies in Medicine* 2000, 8: 32-36 (data provided by ICM Research Ltd)
4 Ong C-K, Banks B. *Complementary and Alternative Medicine: the consumer perspective*. The Prince of Wales's Foundation for Integrated Health, 2003; p13
5 The flight from science. *BMJ* 1980; 280: 1-2
6 Vickers A. Complementary medicine. *BMJ* 2000; 321: 683-686
7 BMA. *Acupuncture: efficacy, safety, and practice*. London: BMA, 2000.
8 *BMJ* 2001; 322
9 Thomas K, Fall M, Parry G, Nichol J. *National survey of access to complementary health care via general practice*. University of Sheffield, Sheffield, 1995.
10 House of Lords Select Committee on Science and Technology. *Complementary and Alternative Medicine. HL Paper 123*. The Stationery Office, London, November 2000
11 Department of Health. *Government Response to the House of Lords Select Committee on Science and Technology's Report on Complementary and Alternative Medicine. CM 5124*. The Stationery Office, 2001

■ The above information is an extract from *Setting the Agenda for the Future*, ISBN 0 9539453 3 2 by The Prince of Wales's Foundation for Integrated Health

Consumer campaign for herbal remedies

Information from the Natural Medicines Society

David Bellamy, world-renowned conservationist and botanist, launched a new campaign as Patron of the consumer charity the Natural Medicines Society, on 11 February 2003. The campaign, HerbA!ert, aims to raise consumer awareness to the needs and concerns facing the future of herbal medicine.

Prof. Bellamy said, 'I am delighted to have been asked to act as a Patron of the Natural Medicines Society to help spearhead a publicity campaign to put herbal medicine back where it deserves to be, an important part of mainstream healing practice in the twenty-first century.'

HerbA!ert aims to provide information to consumers about the herbal products they buy and to steer them to reliable and comprehensive information on medicinal herbs and their use. The campaign will also highlight the need for sustainable harvesting, to ensure long-term availability and campaign to protect the consumer's right to have access to high quality herbal products and treatment from qualified medical herbalists.

With the herbal medicine market in the UK alone being worth in the region of £240 million per year, this campaign is both timely and necessary. Millions of people are choosing herbal remedies every day to cure a variety of ailments from the common cold (Echinacea), cuts (Aloe Vera and Calendula) and bruises (Arnica), right through to the 'modern' illnesses such as mild depression (St John's Wort) and stress (Ginseng). But do consumers really know what is in the herbal product they are buying? And how do they choose from the wide choice on sale?

Due to the massive and fast growth of this market, appropriate regulation is urgently needed to protect consumers, the environment (where the herbs are harvested), practitioners and herbal product manufacturers alike, to ensure the continuation of this most beneficial and traditional healing system.

With the support of Patron David Bellamy, the Natural Medicines Society's HerbA!ert campaign aims to address the key issues of availability, access and regulation – with additional support through individual membership this work will continue, protecting consumer choice, raising essential environmental issues, and fighting for correct legislation.

Michael McIntyre, Chairman of the European Herbal Practitioners' Association, warmly welcomed the initiative from the Natural Medicines Society to improve the quality and safety of herbal medicines. Michael said: 'The increasing popularity of herbal treatment can only be sustained if the public can have absolute confidence in the plant medicines they use and the NMS deserves support and praise for working to ensure that herbal medicines in the UK are of the highest quality.'

■ For further information on the Natural Medicines Society and HerbA!ert visit their web sites at www.the-nms.org.uk and www.herbalert.org.uk

Global strategy

WHO launches the first global strategy on traditional and alternative medicine

Traditional medicine is becoming more popular in the north and up to 80% of people in the south use it as part of primary health care. The situation has given rise to concerns among health practitioners and consumers on the issue of safety, above all, but also on questions of policy, regulation, evidence, biodiversity and preservation and protection of traditional knowledge.

The World Health Organization (WHO) has released a global plan to address those issues. The strategy provides a framework for policy to assist countries to regulate traditional or complementary/alternative medicine (TM/CAM) to make its use safer, more accessible to their populations and sustainable.

'About 80% of the people in Africa use traditional medicine. It is for this reason that we must act quickly to evaluate its safety, efficacy, quality and standardisation – to protect our heritage and to preserve our traditional knowledge. We must also institutionalise and integrate it into our national health systems.' says Ebrahim Samba, WHO's Regional Director for Africa.

In wealthy countries, growing numbers of patients rely on alternative medicine for preventive or palliative care. In France, 75% of the population has used complementary medicine at least once; in Germany, 77% of pain clinics provide acupuncture; and in the United Kingdom, expenditure on complementary or alternative medicine stands at US$ 2300 million per year.

But problems may arise out of incorrect use of traditional therapies. For instance, the herb Ma Huang (ephedra) is traditionally used in China to treat short-term respiratory congestion. In the United States, the herb was marketed as a dietary aid, whose long-term use led to at least a dozen deaths, heart attacks and strokes. In Belgium, at least 70 people required renal transplant or dialysis for interstitial fibrosis of the kidney after taking the wrong herb from the *Aristolochiaceae* family, again as a dietary aid.

'Traditional or complementary medicine is victim of both uncritical enthusiasts and uninformed sceptics,' explains Dr Yasuhiro Suzuki, WHO Executive Director for Health Technology and Pharmaceuticals. 'This strategy is intended to tap into its real potential for people's health and well-being, while minimising the risks of unproven or misused remedies.'

In developing countries, where more than one-third of the population lacks access to essential medicines, the provision of safe and effective TM/CAM therapies could become a critical tool to increase access to health care. But while traditional medicine has been fully integrated into the health systems of China, North and South Korea and Viet Nam, many countries have not collected and standardised evidence on this type of health care.

The global market for traditional therapies stands at US$ 60 billion a year and is steadily growing. In addition to the patient safety issue and the threat to knowledge and biodiversity, there is also the risk that further commercialisation through unregulated use will make these therapies unaffordable to many who rely on them as their primary source of health care. For this reason policies on the protection of indigenous or traditional knowledge are necessary.

About 25% of modern medicines are descended from plants first used traditionally. The efficacy of

---

In wealthy countries, growing numbers of patients rely on alternative medicine for preventive or palliative care

---

acupuncture in relieving pain and nausea has been well established. Randomised controlled trials also offer convincing evidence that therapies such as hypnosis and relaxation techniques can alleviate anxiety, panic disorders and insomnia. Other studies have shown that yoga can reduce asthma attacks while t'ai chi techniques can help the elderly reduce their fear of falls.

As well as addressing chronic conditions, TM can also impact on infectious diseases. In Africa, North America and Europe, three out of four people living with HIV/AIDS use some form of traditional or complementary treatment for various symptoms and conditions. In South Africa, the Medical Research Council is conducting studies on the plant *Sutherlandia microphylla*'s efficacy in treating AIDS patients. Traditionally used as a tonic, this plant may increase energy, appetite and body mass in people living with HIV.

The Chinese herbal remedy *Artemisia annua*, used for almost 2000 years, has recently been found to be effective against resistant malaria and could give hope of preventing many of the 800,000 deaths among children from severe malaria each year.

The WHO TM/CAM strategy aims to assist countries to:
- develop national policies on the evaluation and regulation of TM/CAM practices;
- create a stronger evidence base on the safety, efficacy and quality of the TM/CAM products and practices;
- ensure availability and affordability of TM/CAM, including essential herbal medicines;
- promote therapeutically sound use of TM/CAM by providers and consumers.
- The above information is from the World Health Organization's web site which can be found at www.who.int

© *World Health Organization*

■ Complementary Medicine (CM) includes many different techniques of treating a patient. These are based on systems practised thousands of years ago and can in fact be considered to be the original forms of medicine. (p. 1)

■ Natural medicine is an umbrella term that includes an enormous range of approaches from aromatherapy to visualisation. (p. 4)

■ Acupuncture is a treatment which can relieve symptoms of some physical and psychological conditions and may encourage the patient's body to heal and repair itself, if it is able to do so. (p. 5)

■ Osteopathy is an established recognised system of diagnosis and treatment, which lays its main emphasis on the structural and functional integrity of the body. (p. 6)

■ Chiropractors treat problems with your joints, bones and muscles, and the effects they have on your nervous system. (p. 8)

■ Aromatherapy is the therapeutic use of essential oils to relieve nervous stress, enhance wellbeing, and promote health and vitality. (p. 10)

■ Herbal medicine is the use of plant remedies in the treatment of disease. It is the oldest known form of medicine. (p. 11)

■ Homeopathy is an effective and scientific system of healing which assists the natural tendency of the body to heal itself. It recognises that all symptoms of ill health are expressions of disharmony within the whole person and that it is the patient who needs treatment not the disease. (p. 12)

■ Chinese herbal medicine is one of the great herbal systems of the world, with an unbroken tradition going back to the 3rd century BC. (p. 14)

■ Reflexology is a method of bringing about relaxation, balance and healing through the stimulation of particular points on the feet, or sometimes on the hands. (p. 15)

■ Iridology complements all therapeutic sciences because it provides vital information needed in order to establish the root cause of ailments, revealing the appropriate treatments required. (p. 17)

■ Naturopathic medicine is the field of health care which works with the body's own efforts to allow optimum expression of physiological, mental/emotional, and physical health, given the individual's genetic make-up and environment. (p. 19)

■ Spiritual healing is a completely natural process that helps us achieve better health and a sense of well-being. This is brought about by transmitting healing energies through the person giving the healing to the person receiving the healing. (p. 20)

■ Half of general practices in England now offer patients some access to complementary or alternative medicines. (p. 21)

■ One Briton in five uses complementary medicine, and according to the most recent Mintel survey, one in 10 uses herbalism or homeopathy. Around £130 million is spent on oils, potions and pills every year in Britain, and the complementary and alternative medicine industry is estimated to be worth £1.6 billion. (p. 28)

■ Yoga uses postural, stretching and breathing exercises, meditation and other techniques. (p. 29)

■ Complementary therapies are used alongside conventional medical treatments. Some of them have been scientifically tested and can be useful to help patients relax and cope with stress, pain and side effects of standard cancer treatment. Alternative therapies are more often used instead of conventional medical treatment. (p. 32)

■ 35% of the general public revealed that they take complementary supplements without really understanding what they are supposed to do for them. (p. 35)

■ 52% would buy complementary health products on the back of a newspaper or magazine recommendation. (p. 35)

■ Integrated medicine or healthcare is not another term for complementary medicine, nor does it represent an alternative to conventional care. An integrated approach is much wider. It focuses on health and healing, rather than just disease and treatment and seeks to bring together body, mind and spirit so that healthcare encompasses the whole person. (p. 36)

■ At least 40% of general practices in the UK provide some form of complementary services. (p. 37)

■ In France, 75% of the population has used complementary medicine at least once; in Germany, 77% of pain clinics provide acupuncture; and in the United Kingdom, expenditure on complementary or alternative medicine stands at US$ 2300 million per year. (p. 39)

ADDITIONAL RESOURCES

You might like to contact the following organisations for further information. Due to the increasing cost of postage, many organisations cannot respond to enquiries unless they receive a stamped, addressed envelope.

Association of Reflexologists
27 Old Gloucester Street
London, WC1N 3XX
Tel: 0870 5673320
E-mail: info@aor.org.uk
Web site: www.aor.org.uk

British Chiropractic Association
Blagrave House
17 Blagrave Street
Reading, RG1 1QB
Tel: 0118 950 5950
E-mail: enquiries@chiropractic-uk.co.uk
Web site: www.chiropractic-uk.co.uk

British Medical Acupuncture Society (BMAS)
BMAS House
3 Winnington Court
Northwich, CW8 1AQ
Tel: 01606 786782
Fax: 01606 786783
E-mail: Admin@medical-acupuncture.org.uk
Web site: www.medical-acupuncture.co.uk

Cancer Research UK
PO Box 123
Lincoln's Inn Fields
London, WC2A 3PX
Tel: 020 7242 0200
Fax: 020 7269 3262
E-mail: publications@cancer.org.uk
Web site:
www.cancerresearchuk.org

Complementary Medicine
Peninsula Medical School
Universities of Exeter & Plymouth
25 Victoria Park Road
Exeter, EX2 4NT
Tel: 01392 430802
Fax: 01392 424989
Web site: www.pms.ac.uk/compmed/

General Council and Register of Naturopaths (GCRN)
Goswell House
2 Goswell Road
Street, BA16 0JG

Tel: 01458 840072
Fax: 01458 840075
E-mail: admin@naturopathy.org.uk
Web site: www.naturopathy.org.uk

General Osteopathic Council
Osteopathy House
176 Tower Bridge Street
London, SE1 3LU
Tel: 020 7357 6655
Fax: 020 7357 0011
E-mail: info@osteopathy.org.uk
Web site: www.osteopathy.org.uk

Guild of Naturopathic Iridologists
94 Grosvenor Road
London, SW1V 3LF
Tel: 020 7821 0255
E-mail: info@gni-international.org
Web site: www.gni-international.org

Institute for Complementary Medicine (ICM)
PO Box 194
London, SE16 1QZ
Tel: 020 7237 5165
Fax: 020 7237 5175
E-mail: icm@icmedicine.co.uk
Web site: www.icmedicine.co.uk

International Federation of Professional Aromatherapists
ISPA House
82 Ashby Road
Hinckley, LE10 1SN
Tel: 01455 637987
Fax: 01455 890956
E-mail: admin@ifparoma.org
Web site: www.the-ifpa.org

National Federation of Spiritual Healers
Old Manor Farm Studio
Church Street
Sunbury on Thames, TW16 6RG
Tel: 0845 1232777
Fax: 01932 779648
E-mail: office@nfsh.org.uk
Web site: www.nfsh.org.uk

National Institute of Medical Herbalists
56 Longbrook Street
Exeter, EX4 6AH

Tel: 01392 426022
Fax: 01392 498963
E-mail:
nimh@ukexeter.freeserve.co.uk
Web site: www.nimh.org.uk

Natural Medicines Society (NMS)
PO Box 205
Hampton
Middlesex, TW12 3WP
Tel: 0870 240 4784
E-mail: enquiries@the-nms.org.uk
Web site: www.the-nms.org.uk

Prince of Wales's Foundation for Integrated Health
12 Chillingworth Road
London, N7 8QJ
Tel: 020 7619 6140
Fax: 020 7700 8434
E-mail: info@fihealth.org.uk
Web site: www.fihealth.org.uk

Register of Chinese Herbal Medicine (RCHM)
Office 5, Ferndale Business Centre
1 Exeter Street
Norwich
Norfolk, NR2 4QB
Tel: 01603 623994
Fax: 01603 667447
E-mail: herbmed@rchm.co.uk
Web site: www.rchm.co.uk

Society of Homeopaths
11 Brookfield
Duncan Close, Moulton Park
Northampton, NN3 6WL
Tel: 0845 450 6611
Fax: 0845 450 6622
E-mail: info@homeopathy-soh.org
Web site: www.homeopathy-soh.org

World Health Organization (WHO)
20 Avenue Appia
1211-Geneva 27
Switzerland
Tel: + 41 22 791 2111
Fax: + 41 22 791 3111
E-mail: info@who.ch
Web site: www.who.int

INDEX

ACKNOWLEDGEMENTS

The publisher is grateful for permission to reproduce the following material.

While every care has been taken to trace and acknowledge copyright, the publisher tenders its apology for any accidental infringement or where copyright has proved untraceable. The publisher would be pleased to come to a suitable arrangement in any such case with the rightful owner.

Chapter One: Complementary Medicine

What is complementary medicine?, © Institute for Complementary Medicine (ICM), *What is natural medicine?*, © Saga Magazine, *About acupuncture*, © The British Medical Acupuncture Society (BMAS), *Osteopathy in the UK*, © General Osteopathic Council, *Chiropractic*, © British Chiropractic Association, *Categories of CAM disciplines*, © House of Lords Select Committee Report, 2000, *Professional aromatherapy*, © The International Federation of Professional Aromatherapists, *Herbal medicine*, © National Institute of Medical Herbalists, *Homeopathy simply explained*, © The Society of Homeopaths, *Chinese herbal medicine*, © The Register of Chinese Herbal Medicine, *Popularity of therapies*, © The Prince of Wales's Foundation for Integrated Health, *Reflexology*, © Association of Reflexologists (AoR), *Iridology*, © Guild of Naturopathic Iridologists, *Naturopathy definitions*, © General Council and Register of Naturopaths, *What is spiritual healing and what does it do?*, © National Federation of Spiritual Healers (NFSH), *GPs offer patients complementary medicine*, © BMJ Publishing Group, *Age distribution of users versus non-users of CAM*, © The Prince of Wales's Foundation for Integrated Health.

Chapter Two: The Debate

When there's no real alternative, © Guardian Newspapers Limited 2003, *The alternative professor*, © Guardian Newspapers Limited 2003, *Reasons for using CAM*, © The Prince of Wales's Foundation for Integrated Health, *Hands-on healing, or a con?*, © Telegraph Group Limited, London 2004, *Alternative therapies win NHS backing*, © Guardian Newspapers Limited 2003, *Building confidence in CAM*, © Complementary Medicine at the Universities of Exeter & Plymouth, *Complementary and alternative therapies*, © Cancer Research UK, *Why bogus therapies seem to work*, © Bandolier, *An iguana a day keeps the doctor away?*, © Tesco, December 2003, *Mean expenditure*, © The Prince of Wales's Foundation for Integrated Health, *Setting the agenda for the future*, © The Prince of Wales's Foundation for Integrated Health, *Consumer campaign for herbal remedies*, © The Natural Medicines Society, *Global strategy*, © World Health Organization.

Photographs and illustrations:

Pages 1, 10, 25: Pumpkin House; pages 3, 19, 28, 34: Bev Aisbett, page 4: Angelo Madrid; pages 7, 13, 22, 30, 36: Simon Kneebone.

Craig Donnellan
Cambridge
April, 2004